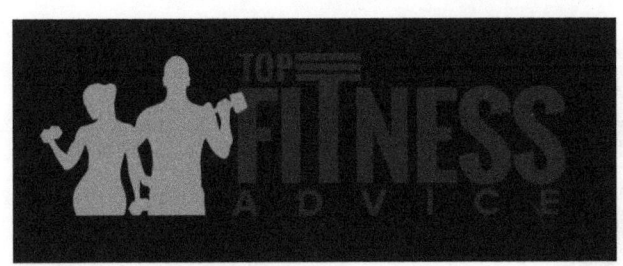

CLEAN EATING

4th Edition

31-Day Clean Eating Meal Plan to Lose Weight & Get Healthy

LINDA WESTWOOD

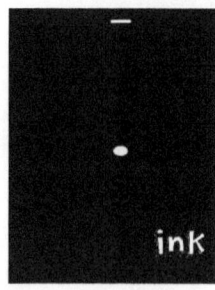

First published in 2015 by Venture Ink Publishing

Copyright © Top Fitness Advice 2019

All rights reserved.

No part of this book may be reproduced in any form without permission in writing from the author. No part of this publication may be reproduced or transmitted in any form or by any means, mechanic, electronic, photocopying, recording, by any storage or retrieval system, or transmitted by email without the permission in writing from the author and publisher.

Requests to the publisher for permission should be addressed to publishing@ventureink.co

For more information about the contents of this book or questions to the author, please contact Linda Westwood at linda@topfitnessadvice.com

Disclaimer

This book provides wellness management information in an informative and educational manner only, with information that is general in nature and that is not specific to you, the reader. The contents of this book are intended to assist you and other readers in your personal wellness efforts. Consult your physician regarding the applicability of any information provided in this book to you.

Nothing in this book should be construed as personal advice or diagnosis, and must not be used in this manner. The information provided about conditions is general in nature. This information does not cover all possible uses, actions, precautions, side-effects, or interactions of medicines, or medical procedures. The information in this book should not be considered as complete and does not cover all diseases, ailments, physical conditions, or their treatment.

You should consult with your physician before beginning any exercise, weight loss, or health care program. This book should not be used in place of a call or visit to a competent health-care professional. You should consult a health care professional before adopting any of the suggestions in this book or before drawing inferences from it.

Any decision regarding treatment and medication for your condition should be made with the advice and consultation of a qualified health care professional. If you have, or suspect you have, a health-care problem, then you should immediately contact a qualified health care professional for treatment.

No Warranties: The author and publisher don't guarantee or warrant the quality, accuracy, completeness, timeliness, appropriateness or suitability of the information in this book, or of any product or services referenced in this book.

The information in this book is provided on an "as is" basis and the author and publisher make no representations or warranties of any kind with respect to this information. This book may contain inaccuracies, typographical errors, or other errors.

Liability Disclaimer: The publisher, author, and other parties involved in the creation, production, provision of information, or delivery of this book specifically disclaim any responsibility, and shall not be held liable for any damages, claims, injuries, losses, liabilities, costs, or obligations including any direct, indirect, special, incidental, or consequences damages (collectively known as "Damages") whatsoever and howsoever caused, arising out of, or in connection with the use or misuse of the site and the information contained within it, whether such Damages arise in contract, tort, negligence, equity, statute law, or by way of other legal theory.

Table of Contents

Disclaimer	3
Introduction	8
Week 1: Day 1	10
Week 1: Day 2	16
Week 1: Day 3	24
Week 1: Day 4	30
Week 1: Day 5	36
Week 1: Day 6	42
Week 1: Day 7	48
Week 2: Day 1	54
Week 2: Day 2	60
Week 2: Day 3	66
Week 2: Day 4	72
Week 2: Day 5	76
Week 2: Day 6	82
Week 2: Day 7	88
Week 3: Day 1	94
Week 3: Day 2	100
Week 3: Day 3	106

Week 3: Day 4	112
Week 3: Day 5	118
Week 3: Day 6	124
Week 3: Day 7	128
Week 4: Day 1	132
Week 4: Day 2	138
Week 4: Day 3	142
Week 4: Day 4	146
Week 4: Day 5	152
Week 4: Day 6	156
Week 4: Day 7	161
Week 5: Day 1	166
Week 5: Day 2	170
Week 5: Day 3	174
Final Words	182

Would you prefer to listen to my book, rather than read it?

Download the audiobook version for free!

If you go to the special link below and sign up to Audible as a new customer, you can get the audiobook version of my book completely free.

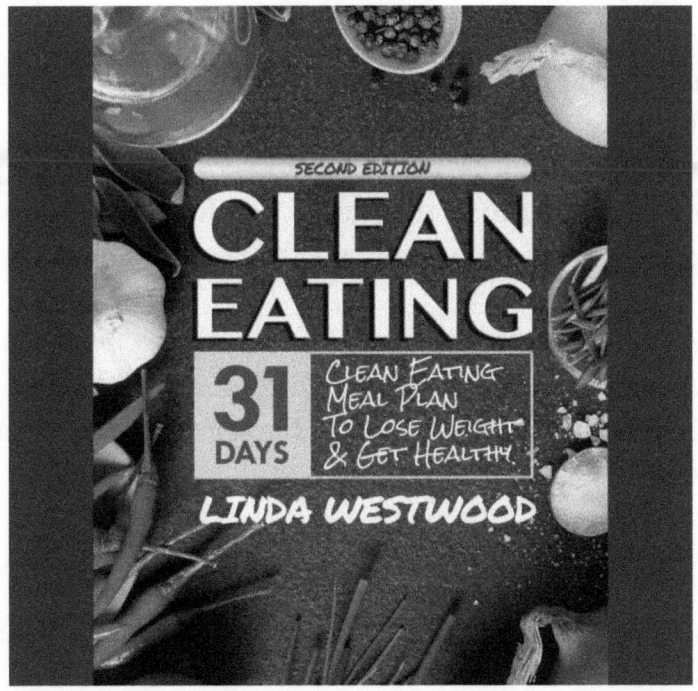

Go here to get your audiobook version for free:

TopFitnessAdvice.com/go/cleaneating

Introduction

The meal plans in this book are aimed at gently propelling you toward healthy eating. It is a common misconception that if you choose to eat healthy you will not eat tasty and delicious food.

The basis of this theory is that food for clean eating is not tasty. The object of this book is, therefore, to dispel that falsehood and show you just how enjoyable eating healthy, clean foods can be.

The basic principles of clean eating differ from theorist to theorist. Some say if it is not from the ground or it has no mother, it should not be eaten. Clean eating for the purpose of this book considers food that keeps you healthy, which means no processed foods and strictly no junk food.

Cooking your own meals ensures you know what is in them and the combination of carbohydrates and proteins in the meals is meant to keep you full longer so that you are not easily tempted.

Happy cooking, and enjoy eating clean.

Week 1

Day 1

Breakfast: Slow Cooker Breakfast Casserole

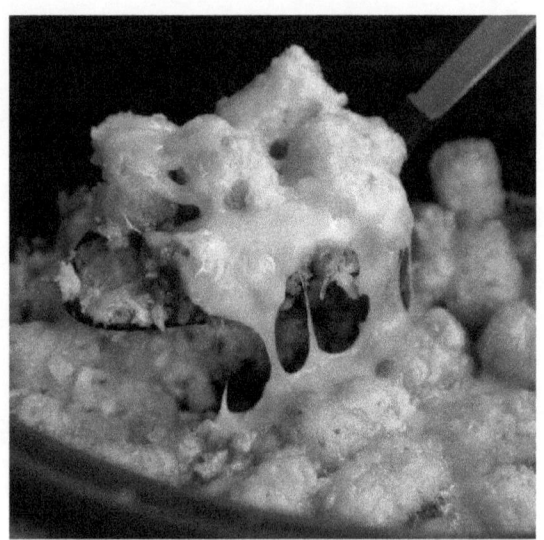

Ingredients

- 8 whole eggs
- 4 egg whites
- ¾ cup milk
- 2 teaspoons ground mustard
- ½ teaspoon garlic salt
- 1 teaspoon salt
- ½ teaspoon pepper
- 1 large bag of frozen hash browns
- ½ onion

- 2 bell peppers
- 1 small head of broccoli
- 6 ounces cheddar cheese

Method

1. In a medium bowl, mix together the first seven ingredients (eggs through pepper). Set the bowl aside for later.

2. Chop up the vegetables. Spray a slow cooker with cooking spray. Place half the hash browns in the slow cooker.

3. Add in half of the bell peppers, onion, broccoli, and cheddar cheese. Cover with the rest of the hash browns. Add the rest of the vegetables and cheddar cheese.

4. Pour the eggs into the slow cooker, over the vegetables and hash browns.

5. Cook for 3-5 hours on low heat.

Lunch: Spicy Fried Chicken

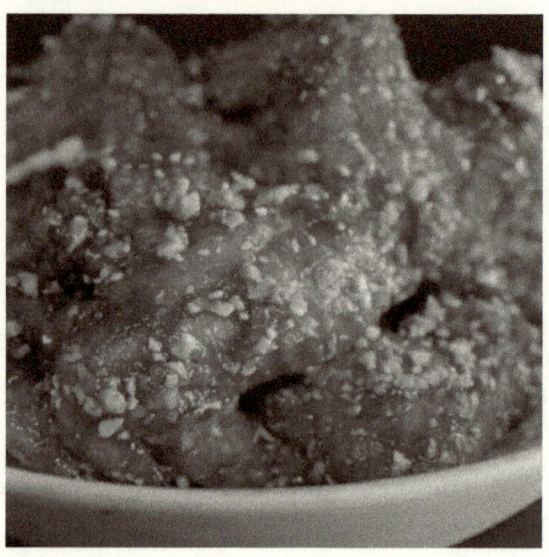

Ingredients

- 2 cups of whole grain cereal (like Kashi or Total)
- 2-4 teaspoons of cajun seasoning
- 1 large egg
- 1-pound chicken breasts (cut into small strips)

Method

1. Preheat the oven to 200 degrees C. In a food processor, pulse the cereal until it is very fine. Pour the cereal into a small bowl and mix in the seasoning.

2. In a separate bowl, whisk the egg. Dip the chicken strips into the egg mixture, and then into the cereal mixture. Place them on a cookie sheet that has been lightly sprayed with cooking spray.

3. Bake the chicken for 15-18 minutes (depending on how thick the strips are). Allow them to cool at least 5 minutes before serving.

Dinner: Lamb & Mushrooms

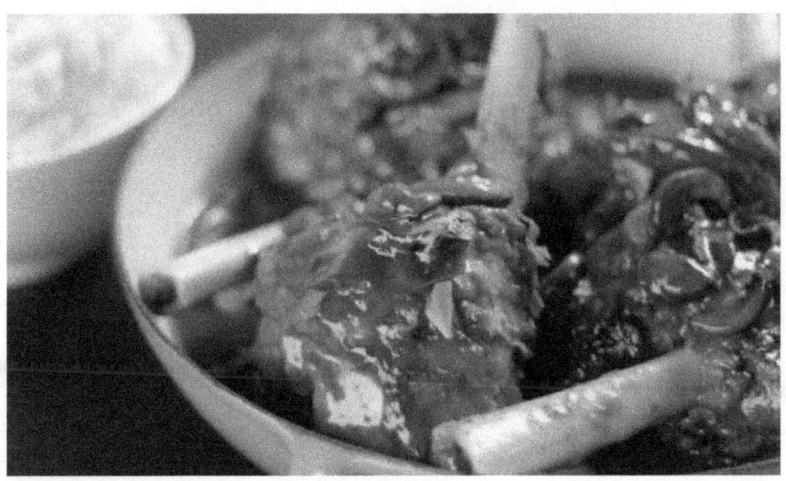

Ingredients

- 1-pound lamb steak (sliced into ½ inch pieces)
- 1 cm long chunk fresh ginger (chopped)
- 12 ounces spring greens (sliced)
- 6 ounces pack sliced mushrooms
- 4 tablespoons oyster sauce
- 2 tablespoons each dark soy sauce and vegetable oil

Method

1. In a small bowl, combine the oyster sauce and soy sauce. Set it aside for later.

2. Heat a skillet to medium-high heat. Add 1 tablespoon of olive oil. Once the oil is hot, add the meat to the skillet. Cook until the lamb is fully cooked. Remove the meat from the pan to rest.

3. Add the remaining oil to the skillet. Stir-fry the ginger until it is golden (just a few seconds).

4. Add in the spring greens and mushrooms. Cook for 2-3 minutes. Add in the steak and sauce mixture. Cook for a few more minutes until the sauce begins to thicken and everything is fully cooked. Serve with boiled potatoes with butter.

Snacks: Peanut Butter Toast & Fruit Smoothie

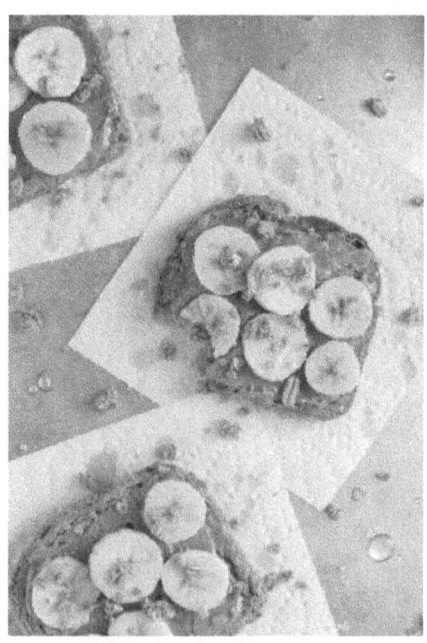

Ingredients

- Whole grain bread
- 2 tablespoons of peanut butter
- Banana
- Soy or almond milk
- Any fruit you like

Method

1. Toast the bread, and spread on 2 tablespoons of peanut butter.

2. Put the banana, milk, and fruit in a blender, and blend until smooth.

Week 1

Day 2

Breakfast: Apple Cinnamon Slow Cooker Oatmeal

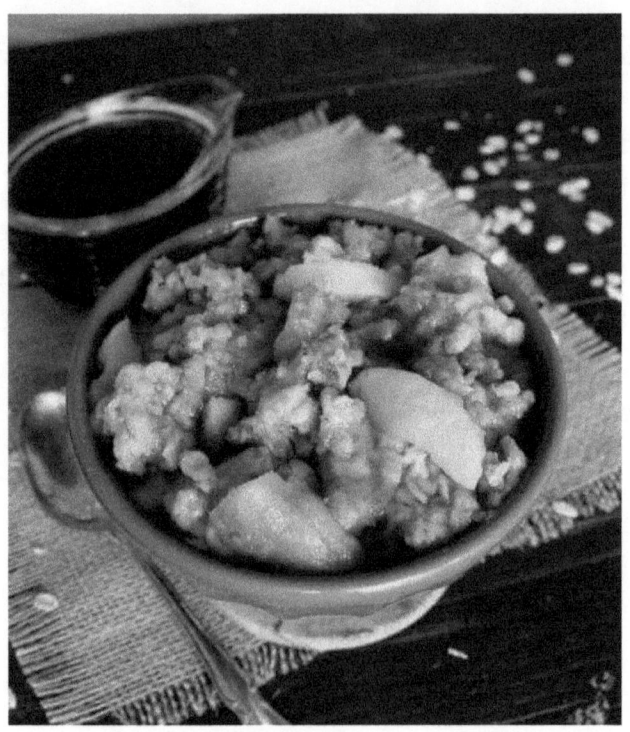

Ingredients

- 2 apples (peeled and cut into bite-sized pieces)
- 1 1/2 cups fat-free milk
- 1 1/2 cups water
- 1 cup steel-cut oats
- 2 tablespoons brown sugar

- 1 1/2 tablespoons butter
- 1/2 teaspoon cinnamon (and more for garnish)
- 1 tablespoon ground flax seeds
- 1/4 teaspoon salt

Method

1. Spray the slow cooker with cooking spray.

2. Add all ingredients to the slow cooker, and cook on low heat overnight (7-8 hours).

3. Serve hot. Garnish with nuts, seeds, cinnamon, or fruit if desired.

Lunch: Chickpea Salad

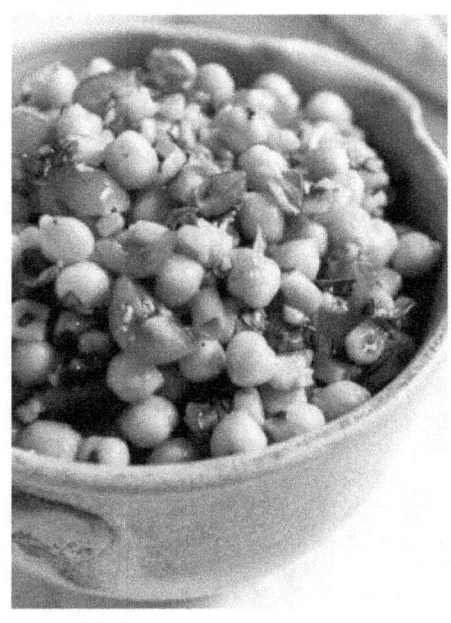

Ingredients

- 1 15-ounce can chickpeas (rinsed and drained)
- 2 tablespoons lemon juice
- 1 clove of garlic (pressed)
- 4 teaspoons extra-virgin olive oil
- 2 tablespoons basil
- 2 tablespoons parsley
- 1/3 cup parmesan cheese
- Salt and pepper to taste

Method

1. In a large bowl, mix together the chickpeas, parsley, basil extra-virgin olive oil, and pressed garlic. Add in the lemon juice, and toss together.

2. Add the Parmesan cheese and toss gently.

3. Season the salad to taste with salt and pepper. You can serve it on its own or wrapped in a tortilla. It tastes best cold, but you can also serve it at room temperature.

Dinner: Slow Cooked Fish Cakes

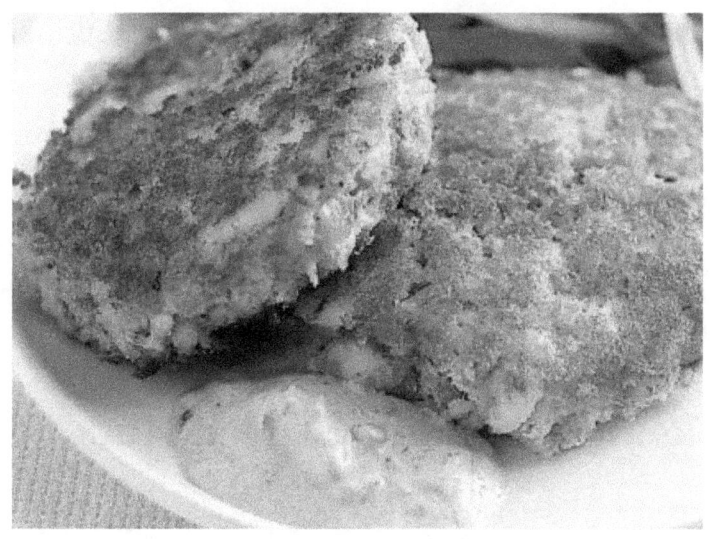

Ingredients

- 1-pound hake steaks
- 2 potatoes (cooked and mashed)
- I onion (grated)
- 3 tablespoons parsley (chopped)
- 2 teaspoons lemon juice
- 2 eggs (beaten)
- 4 tablespoons flour
- Salt and pepper

Method

1. Grease your slow cooker, preferably one with a large base. Put fish into a blender, and blend slightly.

2. Mix fish with mashed potatoes, onions, parsley, lemon juice, eggs, flour, salt, and pepper.

3. Shape the mixture into six small cakes. Sprinkle flour on a board, and roll the fish cakes in the flour.

4. Place the cakes individually into the slow cooker. Close the lid, and cook on low for six hours.

5. Put the fish cakes in the oven, and grill for a minute or two to brown before serving.

Snacks: Fresh Fruit & Dried Nuts

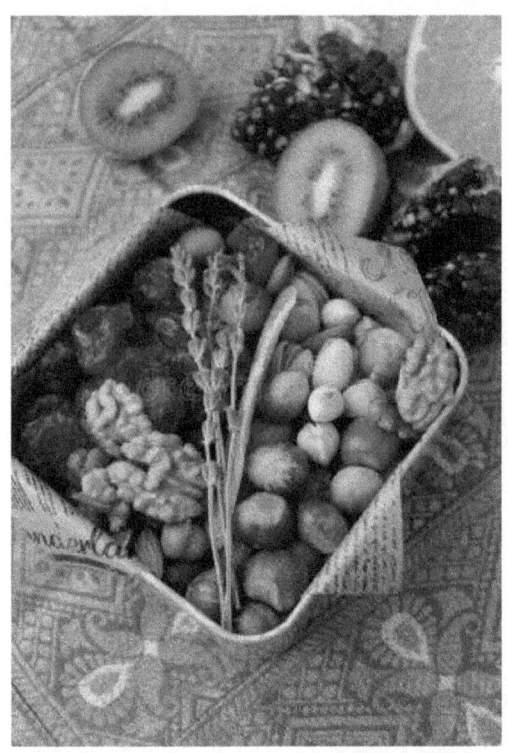

Discover Scientifically-Proven "Shortcuts" & "Hacks" to Lose Weight FASTER (With Very Little Effort)

For this month only, you can get Linda's best-selling & most popular book absolutely free – *Weight Loss Secrets You NEED to Know*.

Get Your FREE Copy Here:
TopFitnessAdvice.com/Bonus

Discover scientifically-proven tips to help you lose weight faster and easier than ever before. With this book, readers were able to improve their weight loss results and fitness levels. So, it's highly recommended that you get this book, especially while it's free!

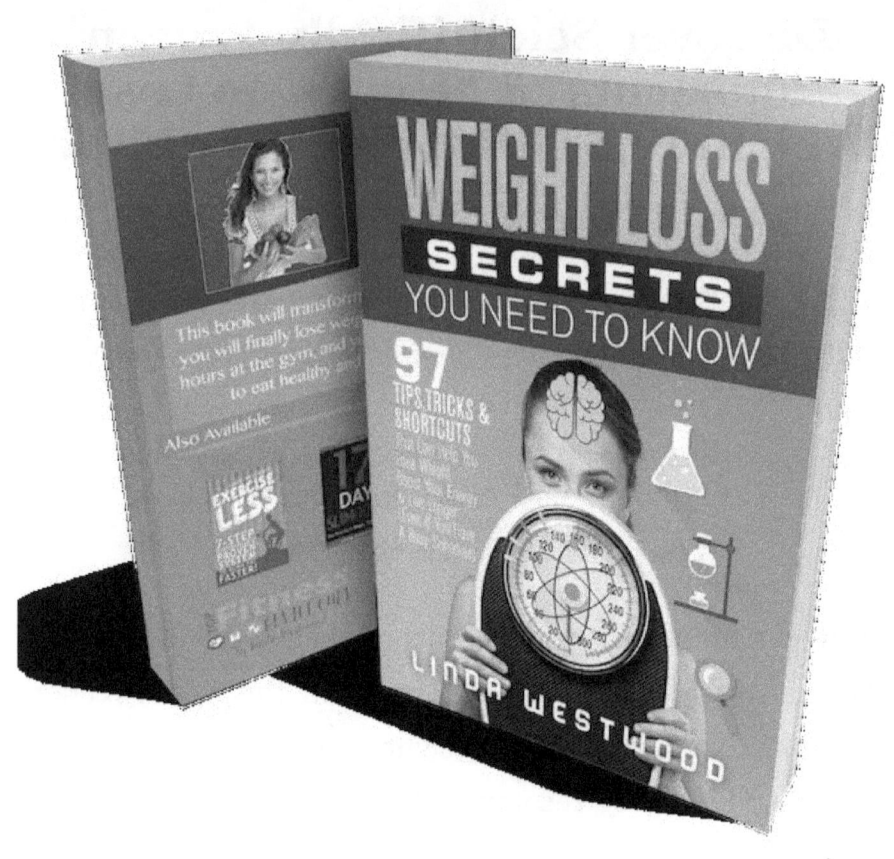

Get Your FREE Copy Here:

TopFitnessAdvice.com/Bonus

Week 1

Day 3

Breakfast: Slow Cooker Chicken Sausage & Egg Casserole

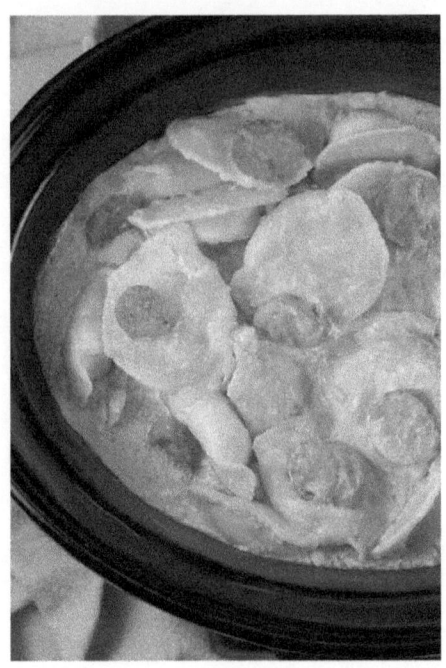

Ingredients

- Cooking spray
- 1 tablespoon olive oil
- 8 large eggs
- ½ cup low fat milk
- ½ cup reduced fat cheddar cheese
- 12-ounce package smoked chicken and apple sausage

- 1 medium sweet potato (peeled and chopped)
- 1 medium red bell pepper (chopped)
- 1 small white onion (peeled and chopped)

Method

1. Spray the slow cooker with cooking spray.

2. Heat the olive oil on medium heat, and add the sausage, sweet potato, bell pepper, and onion until they become tender and slightly translucent.

3. Put the vegetables and sausage into the slow cooker. Whisk together the eggs, milk, and half of the cheddar cheese.

4. Pour the egg mixture over the ingredients in the slow cooker. Cook on low heat for 2-2 ½ hours.

5. Sprinkle remaining cheese over the cooked eggs, and allow the casserole to sit for ten minutes before serving.

Lunch: Crab Salad Stuffed Eggs (Makes 16 Eggs)

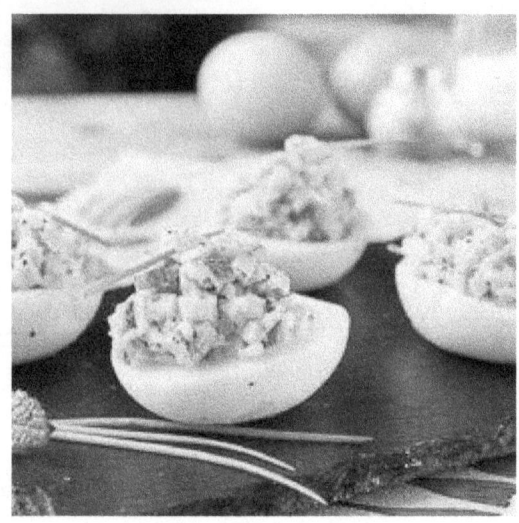

Ingredients

- 2 cups radishes (thinly sliced)
- 1 tablespoon lemon juice
- 1/2 teaspoon salt
- 8 large eggs
- 1/4 teaspoon pepper
- 2 tablespoons extra-virgin olive oil
- 3 tablespoons plain Greek yogurt
- 1 cup crabmeat
- 3 stalks of celery (chopped)
- 1 teaspoon dry mustard

Method

1. In a large bowl, toss together the radishes, lemon juice, and ¼ teaspoon of salt. Cover the bowl and chill in the refrigerator for 30 minutes.

2. Place eggs in a medium pot, and cover them with cold water. The eggs should be submerged b about 1 inch. Bring the water to a boil. Reduce the heat to a simmer for 10 minutes.

3. Place eggs in an ice bath, and let them cool completely. Peel the eggs, and rinse them under cold water. Cut each egg in half. Remove the yolks. Set aside 1 tablespoon of the yolks.

4. Combine remaining 1 teaspoon of lemon juice, remaining yolks, 1/4 teaspoon of salt, and pepper in a small bowl. Slowly pour the oil into the mixture, stirring constantly so everything is combined.

5. Add the yogurt, crabmeat celery, and dry mustard. Stir everything together. Taste the mixture and add more salt or pepper if desired.

6. Stuff the mixture into the centers of the egg whites. One serving is two egg halves.

Dinner: Cauliflower & Broccoli Primavera

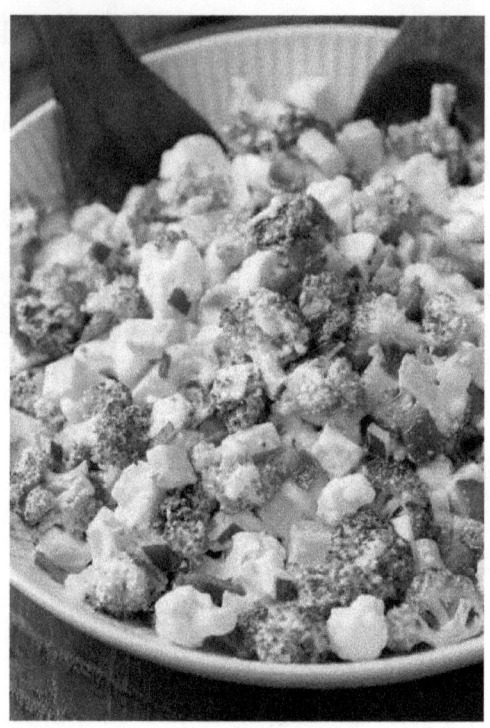

Ingredients

- ¼ cup vegetable oil
- 1-pound cauliflower florets
- 1-pound broccoli floret
- 1-pound sliced carrot
- 18 ounces screws pasta
- ½ cup grated parmesan cheese

Method

1. Boil the pasta according to package instructions, and drain it. In a frying pan, heat the oil on medium heat, and add the vegetables.

2. Season with salt and pepper to taste. Fry for 4 minutes. Be sure not to overcook the vegetables.

3. Add the pasta to the vegetables, and mix well. Sprinkle with cheese, and serve.

Snacks: Any Smoothie & Fresh Vegetables

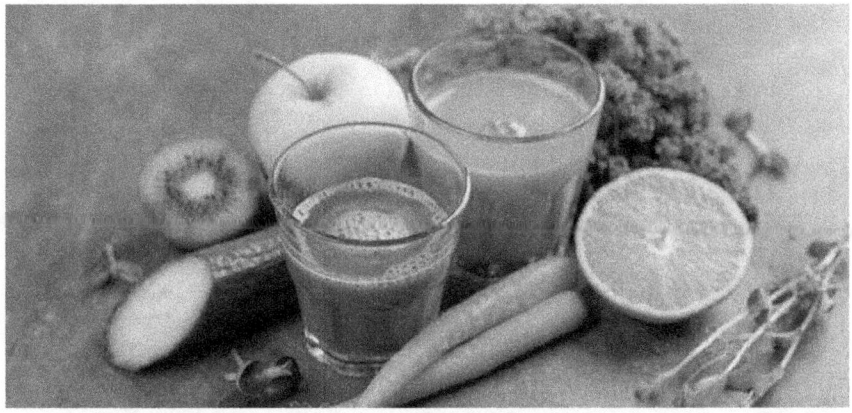

I hope that you are enjoying this book so far, and if you could spare 30 seconds, I would greatly appreciate you leaving a review on Amazon.com.

Week 1

Day 4

Breakfast: Boiled Oats with Banana & Almonds

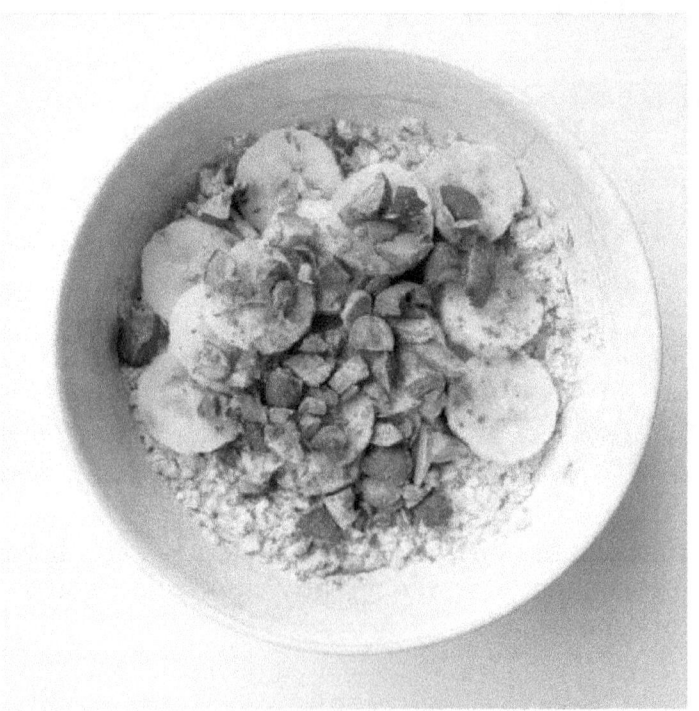

Ingredients

- 1 banana
- 1 tablespoon honey
- 1 teaspoon almond extract
- 1 cup almond milk
- 1/4 teaspoon ground cinnamon

- 1 pinch salt

Method

1. Heat a saucepan on medium-high heat. Mash up half of the banana. Whisk together the honey, almond extract, almond milk, cinnamon, and salt. Combine the mixture with the mashed banana. Add the mixture to the saucepan, and bring to a boil.

2. Stir in the oats. Reduce the heat to a simmer. Cook for about 5-7 minutes until the liquid is absorbed and the oats are as soft as you would like them.

3. Dice remaining half of banana, and put it on top of the oatmeal along with more cinnamon (if desired).

Lunch: Baked Sweet Potato

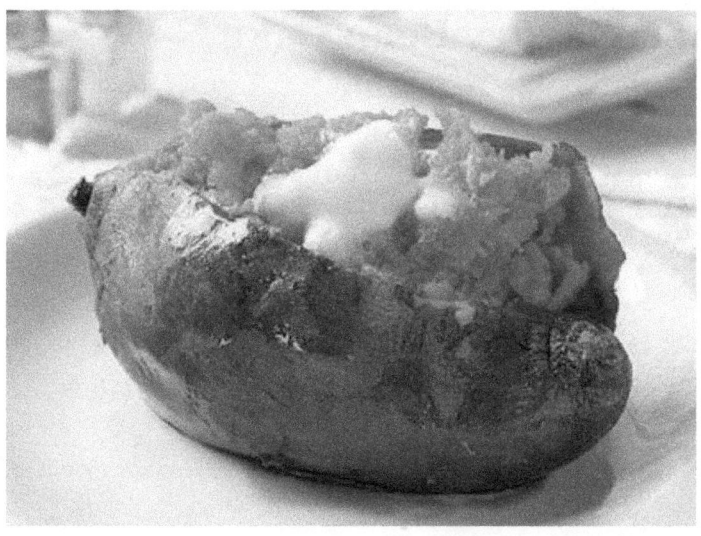

Ingredients

- Large sweet potato
- 1 teaspoon ground cinnamon
- 1 teaspoon of butter

Method

1. Preheat over to 230 degrees C. Thoroughly wash the sweet potato. Wrap it in aluminum foil, and place it in the oven.

2. Bake the potato for 30-40 minutes, until the skin is crisp and the flesh is soft.

3. Remove the potato from the oven. Cut it in half, and coat it with the butter. Sprinkle the cinnamon on the potato, and serve hot.

Dinner: Savory Bean Cake

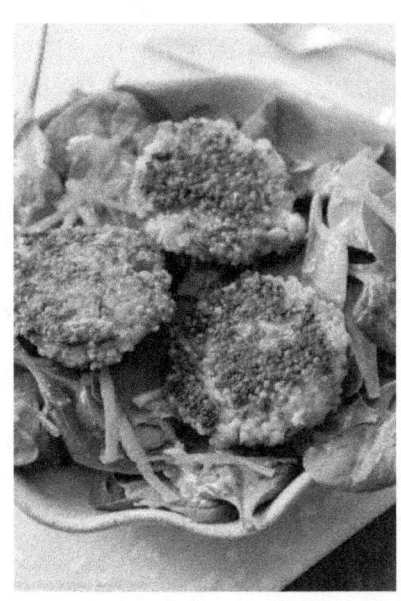

Ingredients

- 3 cups black-eyed beans
- 1 onion (peeled)
- 1 teaspoon curry paste
- 3 tablespoons fresh coriander
- 4 tablespoons butter (melted)
- 1 cup self-raising floor
- 4 eggs (boiled)
- 1 cube chicken stock
- Cooking spray

Method

1. Soak beans for 8-10 hours or overnight. Rinse the beans well, put into blender, and blend until smooth. Remove the beans from the blender.

2. Put onions, pepper, curry paste, stock cube, coriander, and butter into the blender, and blend until smooth

3. Mix the curry blend with the beans. Add flour, and mix again.

4. Spray the slow cooker with cooking spray, and put half the blended mixture on the base.

5. Whisk the eggs. Pour eggs into the slow cooker, and cover them with the rest of the mixture. Close the lid, and cook on low for three hours. Serve with a salad.

Snacks: String Cheese & A Vegetable Smoothie

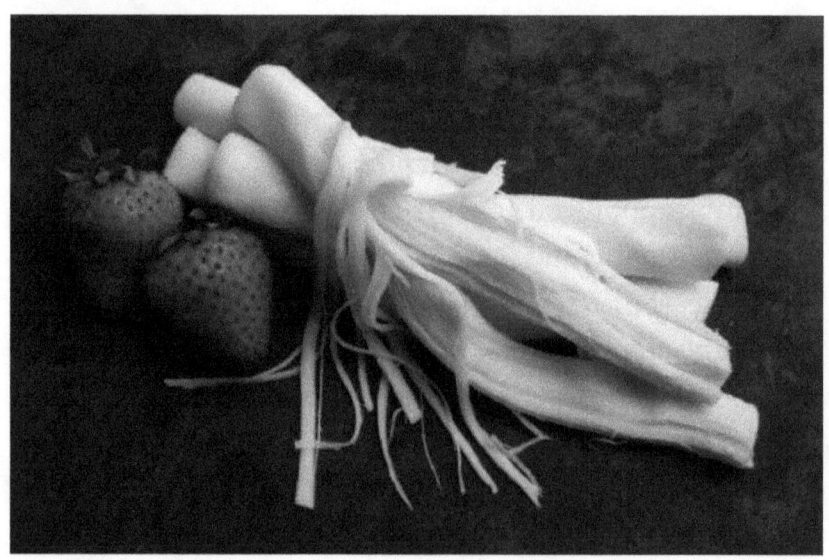

Week 1

Day 5

Breakfast: Tofu Scramble

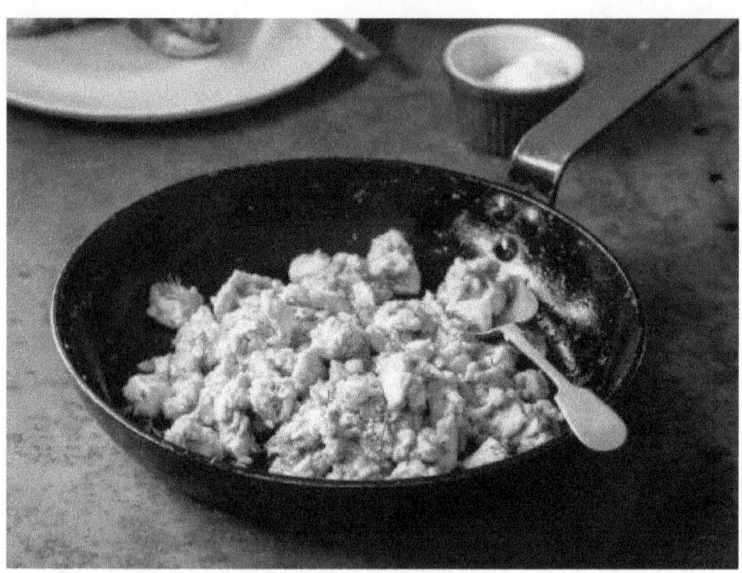

Ingredients

- 8 ounces tofu (extra firm works best, but firm will also work)
- 1-2 tablespoons olive oil
- 1/4 onion (red is best, yellow also works)
- 1/2 red pepper
- 2 cups kale (bitter stem and veins removed)
- 1/2 teaspoon salt
- 1/2 teaspoon garlic powder
- 1/2 teaspoon cumin

- 1/4 teaspoon chili powder
- 1/4 teaspoon turmeric
- Salsa
- Cilantro
- Hot Sauce

Method

1. Use paper towels to remove some of the water form the tofu. Wrap it in a clean towel to absorb as much liquid as possible. Then place the tofu on a plate lined with paper towels to absorb any additional water. (This process will take a few minutes).

2. Add the salt, garlic powder, cumin, chili powder, and turmeric to a small bowl. Add 2-3 tablespoons of water (enough to form a sauce). Heat a large skillet over medium heat. Add the olive oil. Once the olive oil is hot, add the chopped onion and red pepper.

3. Season them with a bit of salt and pepper (as desired) and allow to cook until the onion becomes slightly translucent (about 5 minutes). Add the kale. Season it with salt and pepper, and cover it. Let it steam for about 2 minutes.

4. While this is cooking, crumble the tofu into bite sized pieces. Push the vegetables to one side of the skillet, and add the tofu to the other side. Cook for 2 minutes, and pour the sauce over the vegetables and the tofu.

5. Cook a few more minutes, and then gently toss the tofu and vegetables together. Cook for another 5-7 minutes until the tofu is cooked (it will be slightly brown). Top with hot sauces, cilantro, or salsa.

Lunch: Spicy Fried Chicken

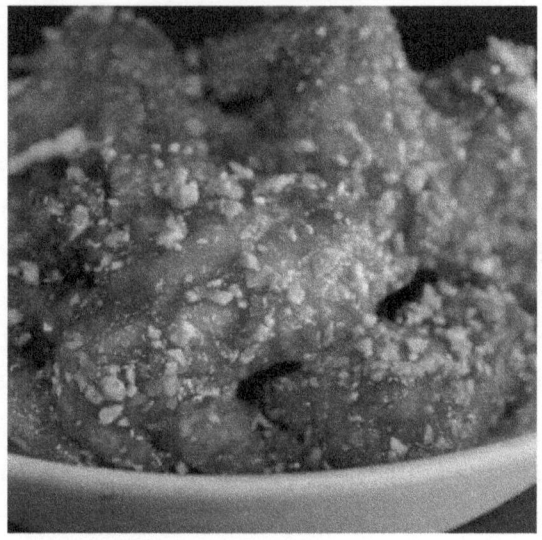

See Week 1 Day 1 For Recipe

Dinner: Slow Cooked Thai Curry Beef with Whole Wheat Pasta

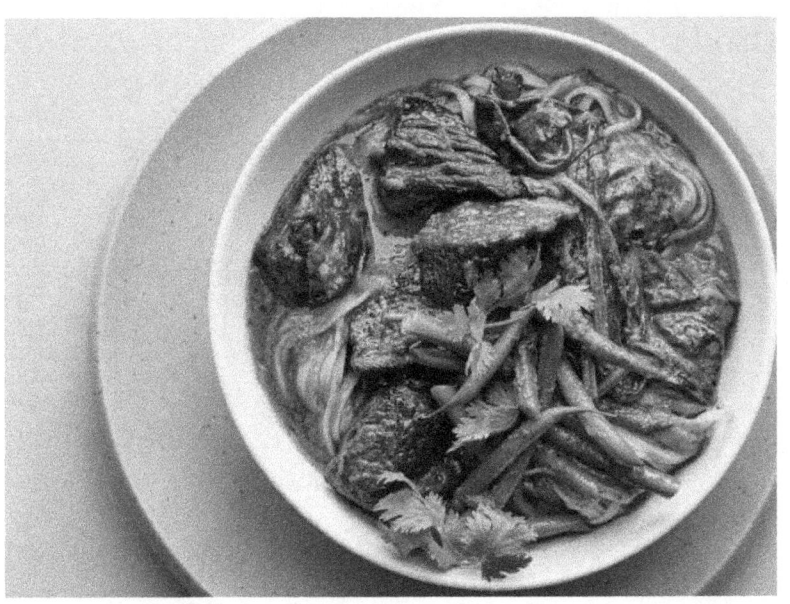

Ingredients

- 4 teaspoons Thai curry paste (red or green, depending on your preference)
- 2 pounds steak (cut into bite-sized pieces)
- 8 ounces mushrooms
- Medium onion
- Medium carrot
- 14 ounce can coconut milk
- 3 tablespoons soy sauce
- 10 ounces cauliflower florets
- 2 teaspoons salt
- ½ teaspoon pepper
- 12 ounces green beans (trimmed and cut into ½ inch pieces)
- Whole wheat pasta

Method

1. Inside a slow cooker, mix together the curry paste, milk, and soy sauce.

2. Add the remaining ingredients (except beans), and stir until everything is fully coated. Add the beans. Don't mix them in.

3. Cook on low heat for 8 hours. In the last 30 minutes, stir in the beans at ten-minute intervals. Serve with boiled whole-wheat pasta.

Snacks: Low Fat Yogurt & A Fresh Apple

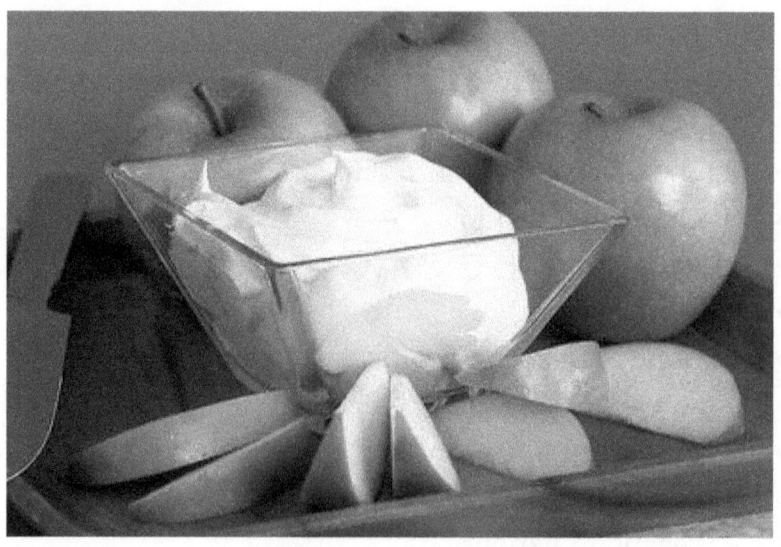

Week 1

Day 6

Breakfast: Oatmeal Porridge

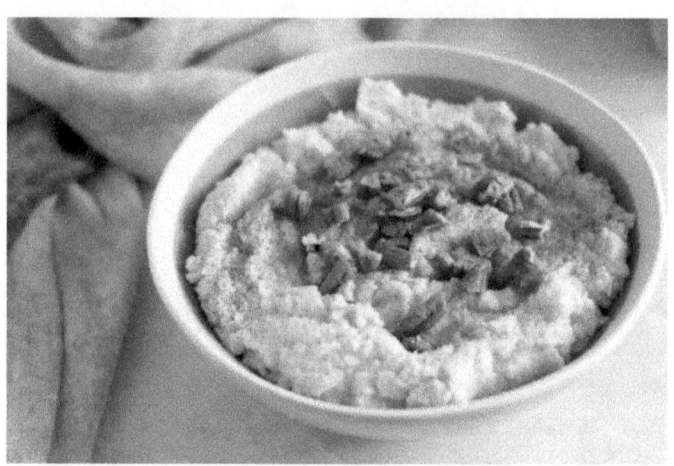

Ingredients

- ½ cup rolled oats (or quick cooking oats if you desire)
- 2 cups water
- ½-1 cup of milk
- 2 tablespoons sugar (or add to taste)
- Dried fruit, nuts, or honey (optional)

Method

1. Put the oats in a pan. Add water and milk. Add more milk if you like your oatmeal a bit thinner, and less milk if you prefer thick oatmeal.

2. Add however much sugar you would like. Stir together and heat the mixture on medium-low heat. Cook for 5-6 minutes, stirring frequently.

3. Serve porridge hot or cold. You can add fruit, nuts, or honey if desired.

Lunch: Vegetable Hash with Boiled Eggs

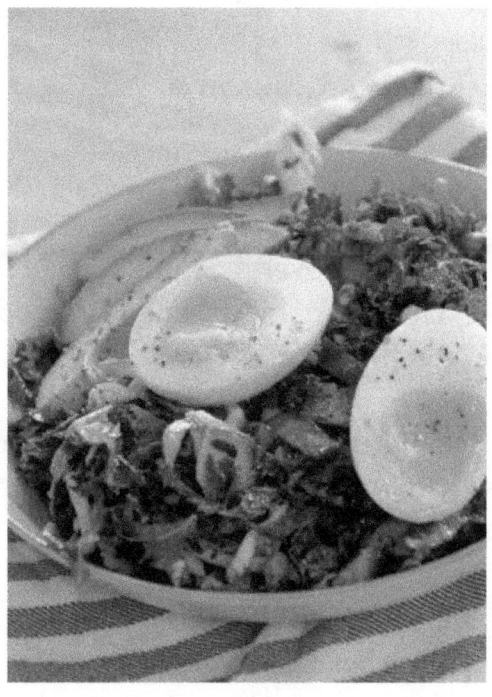

Ingredients

- 4 teaspoons olive oil
- 1 cup sweet onion
- 1 cup small red or fingerling potatoes
- 1 teaspoon dried herbs de Provence

- 1 cup zucchini
- 1 cup yellow squash
- 1 cup green beans (cut into ½ inch pieces)
- 1/2 teaspoon salt
- 1/2 teaspoon pepper (divided)
- 2 cups seeded tomato
- 2 tablespoons chives
- 2 tablespoons fresh flat-leaf parsley
- 1 tablespoon white vinegar
- 4 large eggs
- 1-ounce shredded parmesan cheese

Method

1. Heat a large skillet over medium-high heat, and add the olive oil. Once the oil is very hot, add the onion, potatoes, and herbs de Provence.

2. Spread the mixture in a thin layer in the pan. Cook for 4 minutes, without stirring, or until potatoes are lightly browned.

3. Reduce the heat to medium. Stir in the zucchini, squash, green beans, salt, and 3/8-teaspoon pepper. Cook for about 3 minutes. Remove the pan from the heat. Stir in the tomato, chives, and parsley.

4. Add water to a different skillet, filling two-thirds full; bring to a boil. Reduce heat and bring the water to a simmer. Stir in the vinegar. Carefully break each egg into the water, and use a plastic or metal spoon to push

the white toward the yolk as it cooks. Poach each egg for 2-3 minutes (until they reach the firmness you desire).

5. Carefully remove the eggs from the pan using a slotted metal spoon. Place ¼ of the vegetable mixture on a plate. Top with a boiled egg, and sprinkle with the shredded cheese and pepper.

Dinner: Broiled Tilapia Parmesan

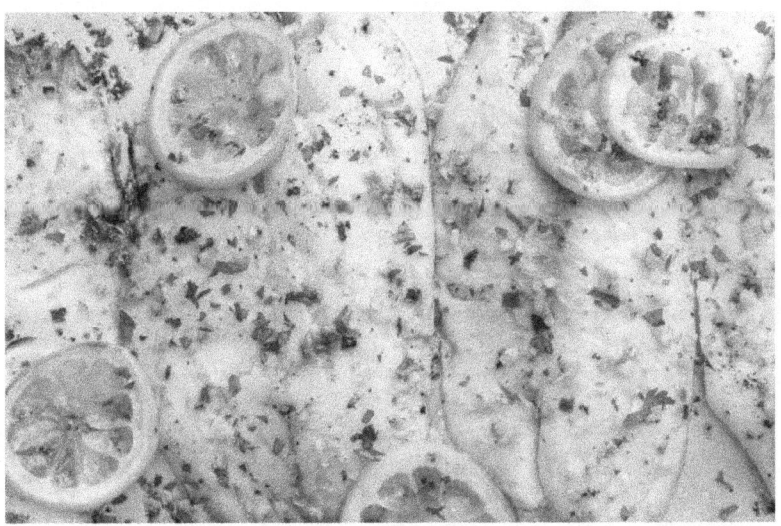

Ingredients

- ¼ cup parmesan cheese
- 2 tablespoons each of butter and mayonnaise
- 1 tablespoon lemon juice
- $1/8$ teaspoon each of dried basil, celery salt, onion powder and ground black pepper
- 1-pound tilapia fillets

Method

1. Preheat the broiler and spray it with cooking spray. Mix all ingredients, except for the fish, in a bowl. Arrange the fillets in a single layer in the pan. Broil them for 3 minutes. Flip them over, and broil for another 3 minutes. Remove fish from the oven.

2. Mix the butter or mayonnaise, lemon juice, herbs, and cheese in a bowl. Sprinkle the cheese mixture on top of the fillets.

3. Broil until topping is browned and fish flakes easily. Remove and serve with mashed potatoes.

Snacks: Peanuts with Raisins & Fresh Fruit Smoothie

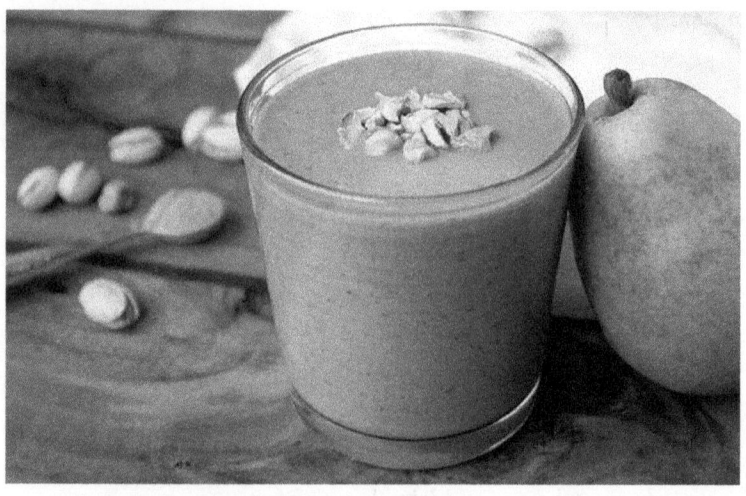

See Week 1 Day 1 For Smoothie Recipe

Week 1

Day 7

Breakfast: Waffles & A Fruit Smoothie

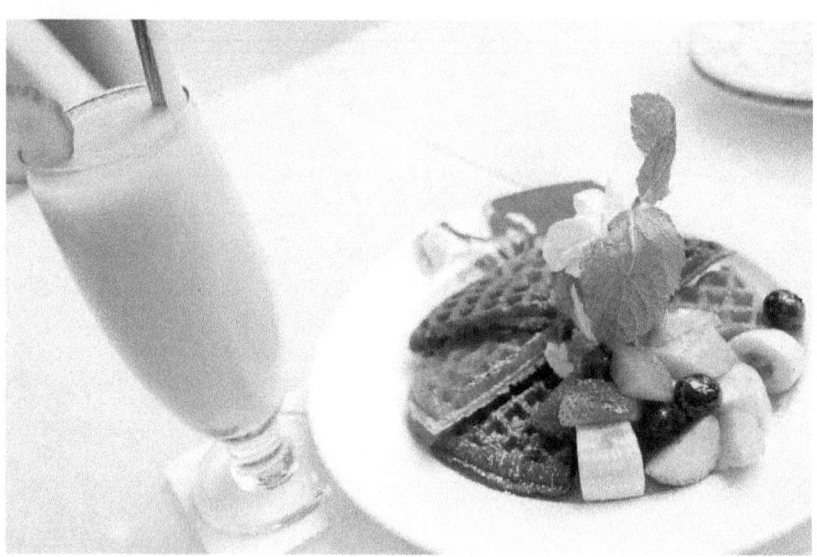

Ingredients

- 2 tablespoons whole wheat flour
- ½ teaspoon baking soda
- ¼ teaspoon ground cinnamon
- ⅛ teaspoon sea salt
- ⅔ cup raw cashews
- 2 large eggs
- ⅓ cup unsweetened almond milk
- ¼ teaspoon vanilla extract
- 2 tablespoons honey
- 2 tablespoons melted coconut oil

- Cooking spray

Method

1. Preheat your waffle maker. In a small bowl, mix together the flour, baking soda, cinnamon, and salt.

2. In a blender, add the cashews, eggs, almond milk, vanilla extract, honey, and coconut oil. Blend them until the mixture is creamy.

3. Add the bowl of dry ingredients to the blender, and again blend it until everything is creamy. Coat the waffle maker with coconut oil

4. Pour a small dollop of the batter into the waffle maker. Cook for about 1 minute.

5. Once the waffle is finished, top it with syrup, butter, powdered sugar, or anything else you desire.

See Week 1 Day 1 For Smoothie Recipe

Lunch: Chicken With Brussels Sprouts & Mustard Sauce

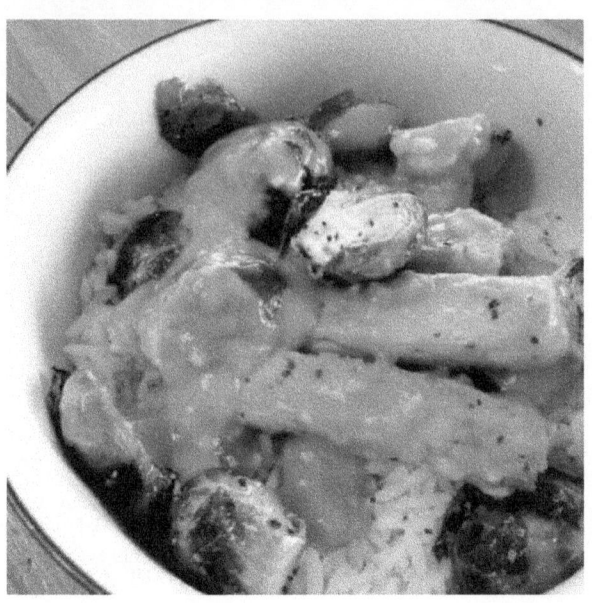

Ingredients

- 2 tablespoons olive oil
- 1/4 cup apple cider
- 2 tablespoons whole-grain Dijon mustard
- 2 tablespoons butter
- 1 tablespoon fresh parsley
- 4 skinless (boneless chicken breast halves)
- 3/8 teaspoon salt
- 1/4 teaspoon pepper
- 3/4 cup chicken stock
- ¾ pound Brussels sprouts (trimmed and halved)

Method

1. Preheat oven to 230 degrees C. Heat a large skillet over high heat. Add 1 tablespoon of olive oil. Coat the

chicken with ¼ teaspoon of salt and ¼ teaspoon of pepper

2. Add the chicken to the hot skillet, and cook for about 3 minutes on each side. Move the skillet to the oven, and cook for 8-10 minutes until it is fully cooked.

3. Remove the chicken form the skillet, and set it aside to rest. Put the skillet back on the stove on medium-high heat. Add 1/2 cup of chicken stock and the apple cider, and bring to a boil.

4. Reduce the heat to medium-low, and allow to simmer for about 4 minutes (until the mixture starts to thicken). Add the mustard, 1 tablespoon of butter, and parsley.

5. Heat remaining olive oil and butter in a large skillet over medium-high heat. Add the Brussels sprouts, and sauté for 2 minutes, or until they are lightly browned.

6. Add in the remaining salt and chicken stock to the pan. Cook for 4 minutes, or until the Brussels sprouts are crispy on the outside and tender. Serve the Brussels sprouts with the chicken.

Dinner: Venetian Style Pasta

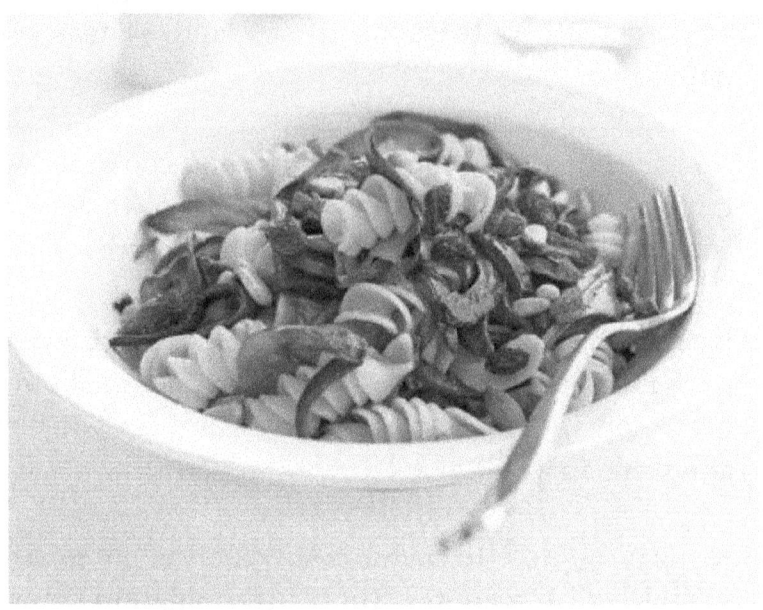

Ingredients

- 2 onions (sliced)
- 1 tablespoon canola oil
- 8 ounces pasta screws
- 4 teaspoon balsamic vinegar
- 2 tablespoon each raisins and toasted pine nuts
- 5 ounces spinach (chopped)

Method

1. Boil pasta for 8-10 minutes. Put oil in a pan and fry the onions until they are slightly brown.

2. Stir in vinegar, raisins, capers, and most of the nuts, and cook for 2 minutes.

3. Stir in the spinach with a little water. Toss the drained pasta with the mixture. Scatter remaining nuts on top of the pasta.

Snacks: String Cheese & Pineapple Tidbits

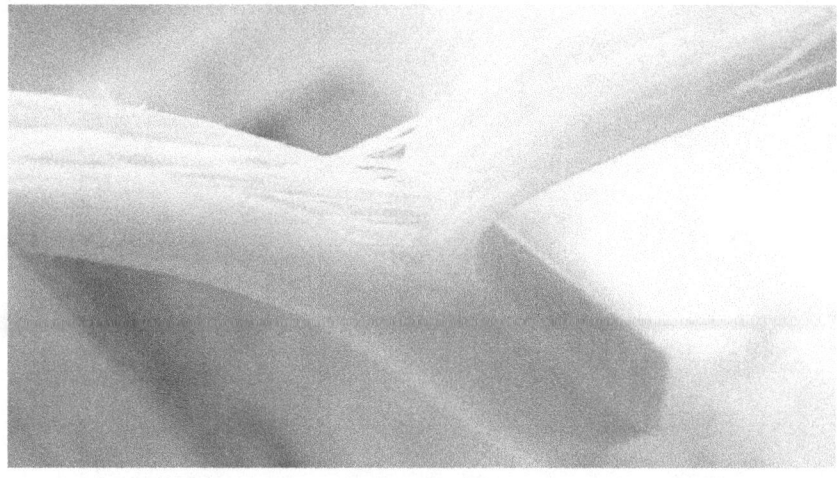

Week 2

Day 1

Breakfast: Homemade Yogurt with Strawberries & Granola

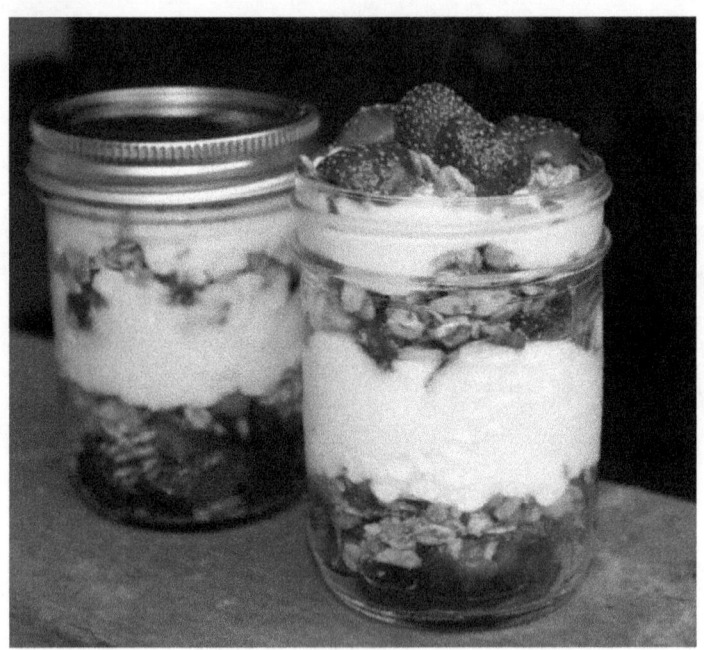

Ingredients

- Fresh strawberries (about a handful)
- 2 tablespoons of granola
- 4 cups whole milk
- 3 tablespoons fresh yogurt starter (from a previous batch or the store)
- 1/3 cup sugar, maple syrup, or honey

- 2 ½ teaspoons vanilla extract
- Pinch of nutmeg or cinnamon

Method

1. Preheat the oven to 43 degrees C. Heat milk in a pot over medium-high heat. Remove from the heat.

2. Reduce the heat to medium-low. Add the fresh yogurt culture to the warm milk. Let it rest 5 minutes, the stir it together gently.

3. Add the sugar, honey, or vanilla. Mix everything together until the sugar dissolves completely. Pour the mixture into a glass jar, and cover with something opaque. Place the jar in the oven, and leave for 6-8 hours.

4. Remove from the oven. Allow it to cool to room temperature (to prevent the hot glass from shattering), and place it in the fridge until it's ready to use.

5. Serve the cold yogurt with strawberries and granola.

Lunch: Boiled Egg & Avocado Whole Wheat Bread Sandwich

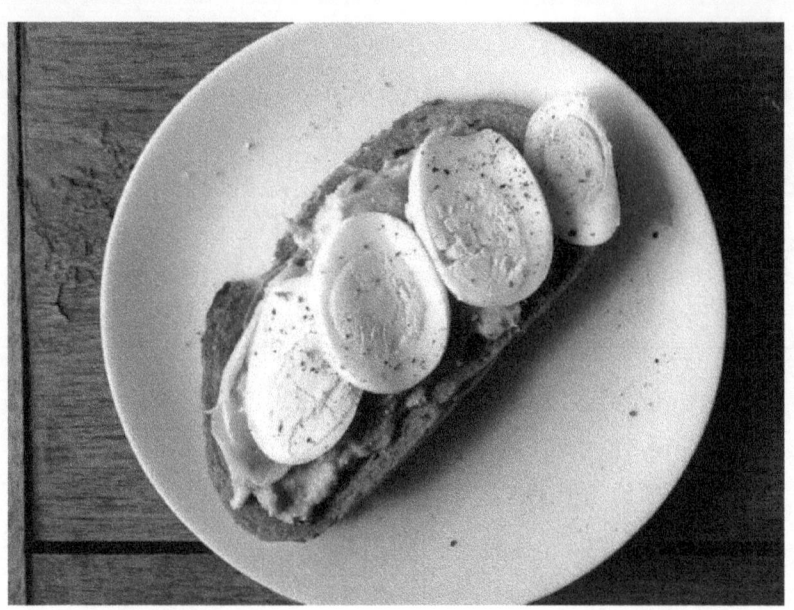

Ingredients

- 2 eggs
- ½ avocado
- 2 pieces of whole wheat bread
- 1 tablespoon light mayonnaise

Method

1. Bring a pot of water to a boil and carefully crack the eggs in to poach them.

2. Remove the eggs after 2-3 minutes, and place them on a plate with a paper towel to drain. Mash up the avocado in a bowl.

3. Spread the mayonnaise and mashed avocado on the pieces of bread. Place the eggs on one half, and put the two slices together.

Dinner: Tandoori Chicken

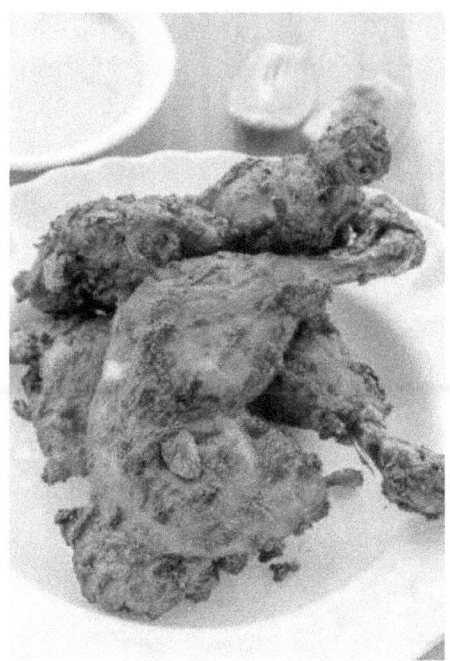

Ingredients

- 1 cup, thick and plain yogurt
- 1 garlic clove (crushed)
- 1 piece peeled and grated ginger
- 1 tablespoon each of lemon juice and olive oil
- 1 teaspoon each of masala and ground coriander
- ½ teaspoon each of chili powder and turmeric
- 6 chicken thigh fillets (trimmed)

Method

1. Mix the yogurt, ginger, garlic, lemon juice, spices, oil, and salt in a large bowl.

2. Double slit the top of each chicken thigh without cutting all the way through. Coat the chicken pieces in the yogurt mixture. Refrigerate for 3½ hours.

3. Preheat the oven to 220 degrees C. Place chicken in a lined dish, and roast until it is thoroughly cooked. Serve with a side of rice.

Snacks: Pear, Roasted Peanuts, & Raisins

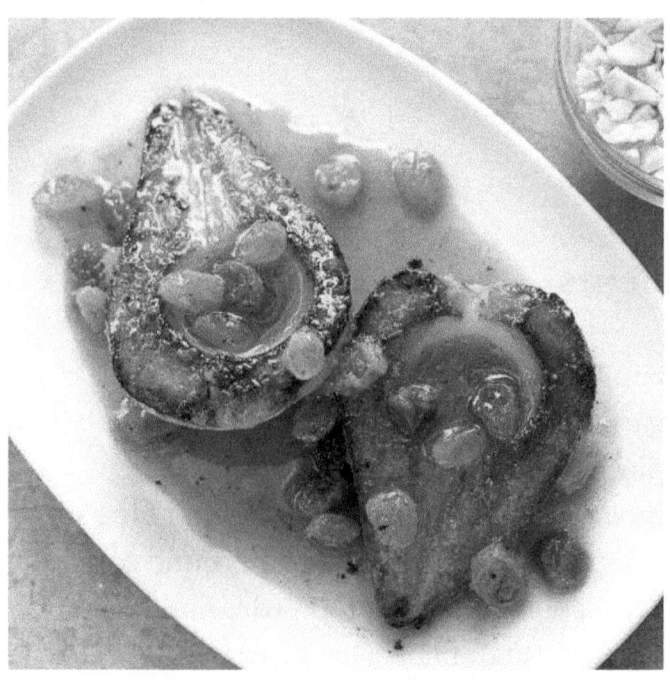

Week 2

Day 2

Breakfast: Whole Wheat Pancakes & A Smoothie

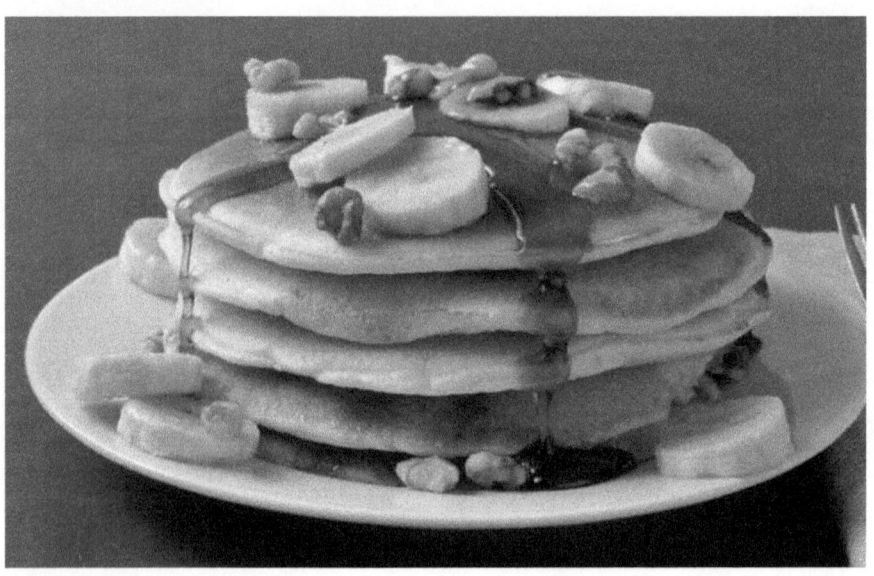

Ingredients

- 1 cup whole wheat flour
- 1/2 cup quick oats
- 1/4 teaspoon salt
- 2 teaspoons baking powder
- 1 teaspoon ground cinnamon
- 1 large egg
- 1 cup milk
- 2 Tablespoons packed dark brown sugar

- 1/4 cup Greek yogurt
- 1 teaspoon vanilla extract
- Additional ingredients if desired (berries, nuts, banana slices, etc.)

Method

1. Heat a skillet to medium-high heat. In a large bowl, combine the whole-wheat flour, quick oats, salt, baking powder, and cinnamon.

2. In a medium bowl, whisk together the egg and milk. Add the brown sugar and yogurt. Stir until everything is smooth. Whisk in the vanilla, and stir again.

3. Make a well in the dry ingredients and pour the wet ingredients into it. If you wish to add any additional ingredients (blueberries, nuts, banana, etc., add them in now)

4. Drop the batter onto the hot skillet in ¼ cup increments. Cook for about 1 minute on each side (until bubble begin to form in the pancake).

5. Serve immediately with butter, syrup, or desired toppings.

See Week 1 Day 1 For Smoothie Recipe

Lunch: Green Salad with Eggs & Vegetables

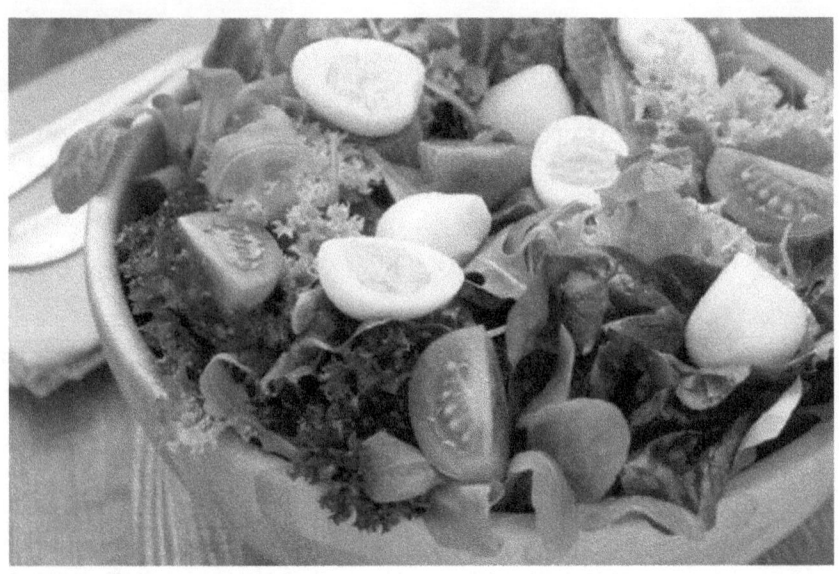

Ingredients

- 2 hardboiled eggs
- Vegetables of your choice (chopped)
- Romaine lettuce
- 2 tablespoons of low-fat dressing

Method

1. Combine all fresh ingredients, and toss them in the dressing.

Dinner: Chicken Curry with Brown Rice

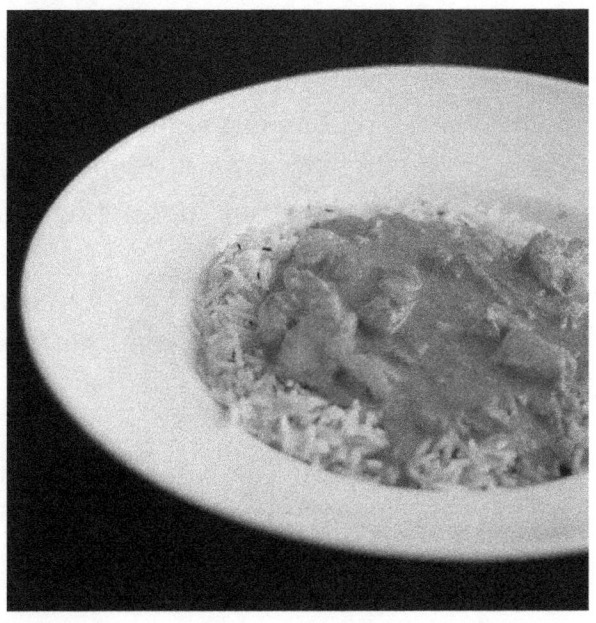

Ingredients

- 2 pounds rinsed chicken pieces
- 2 teaspoon ground ginger and garlic paste
- 1 teaspoon cumin seeds
- 1 cinnamon stick (broken in half)
- 2 cardamom pods
- 2 halves green chili
- 1 aniseed
- 2 teaspoon each of medium hot masala and garam masala
- ½ teaspoon turmeric
- 2 large tomatoes (chopped)
- 3 large potatoes (chunked)
- ½ cup peas
- ½ tablespoon olive oil

Method

1. Slightly brown the onions in the oil. Add cumin, cloves, aniseed, cardamom, cinnamon, and chili. Stir the ingredients together, and cook for another 4 minutes.

2. Reduce the heat to medium, and add the turmeric and masala, stirring for ten seconds. Add tomatoes and cook for 2 minutes.

3. Add the chicken, and use the gravy to coat them as you cook for another 10 minutes. Lower the heat slightly, and add the potatoes, water, and salt.

4. Partially cover the pan, and cook for 20 minutes, stirring frequently. Uncover the pan and cook for 10 more minutes. Add garam masala and peas, and cook together for 5 minutes. Serve with the brown rice.

Snacks: String Cheese & Kale Apple Smoothie

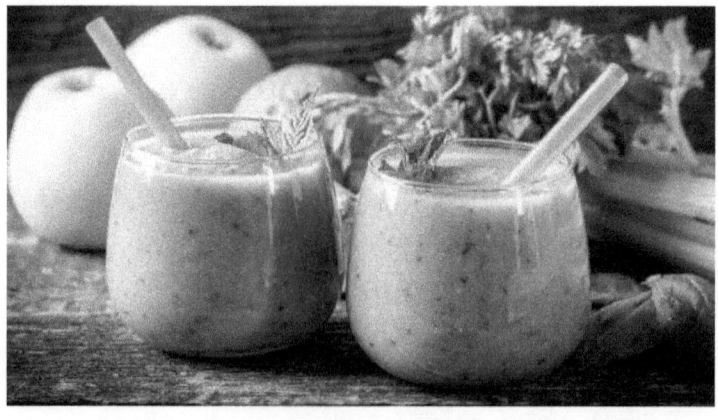

Ingredients (For Smoothie)

- ¾ cup chopped kale
- ½ cup apple juice
- 1 tablespoon fresh lemon juice
- 1 small stalk celery
- ½ banana
- ½ cup ice

Method

1. Remove the stem and veins from the kale. These are very bitter and will ruin the smoothie.

2. Add all ingredients to a blender, and blend until everything is smooth.

Week 2

Day 3

Breakfast: Poached or Boiled Eggs, Toast, & A Smoothie of Your Choice

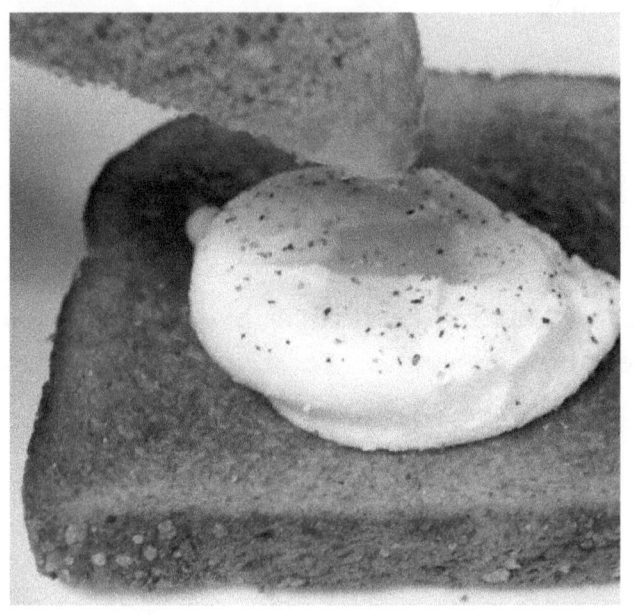

See Week 1 Day 1 For Smoothie Recipe

Lunch: Taco Salad

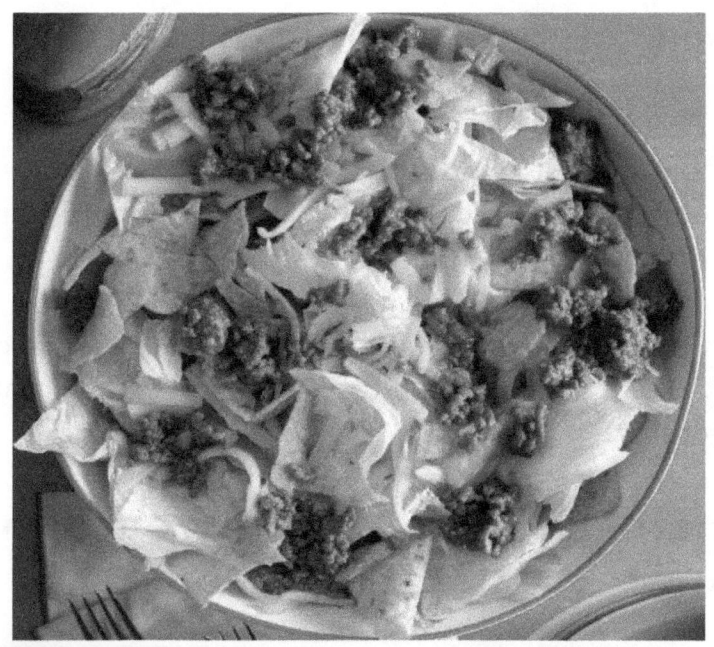

Ingredients

- 12 ounces of ground turkey
- 1 medium sweet red pepper
- 1 small sweet yellow pepper
- 1/3 cup onion (chopped)
- 3 garlic cloves (minced)
- 1 tablespoon olive oil
- 1 ½ cups of salsa
- ½ cup kidney beans (drained and rinsed)
- 2 teaspoons chili powder
- 1 teaspoon ground cumin
- 8 cups torn romaine
- 2 tablespoons fresh cilantro (for garnish)

Method

1. Heat a large skillet to medium-high heat. Add olive oil to the pan. Once the oil is hot, add the turkey, peppers, onion, and garlic. Cook for about 6 minutes until the turkey is cooked through.

2. Stir in the salsa, kidney beans, chili powder, and cumin. Serve over romaine lettuce, and top with the cilantro if desired.

Dinner: Grilled Salmon & Boiled Sweet Potato

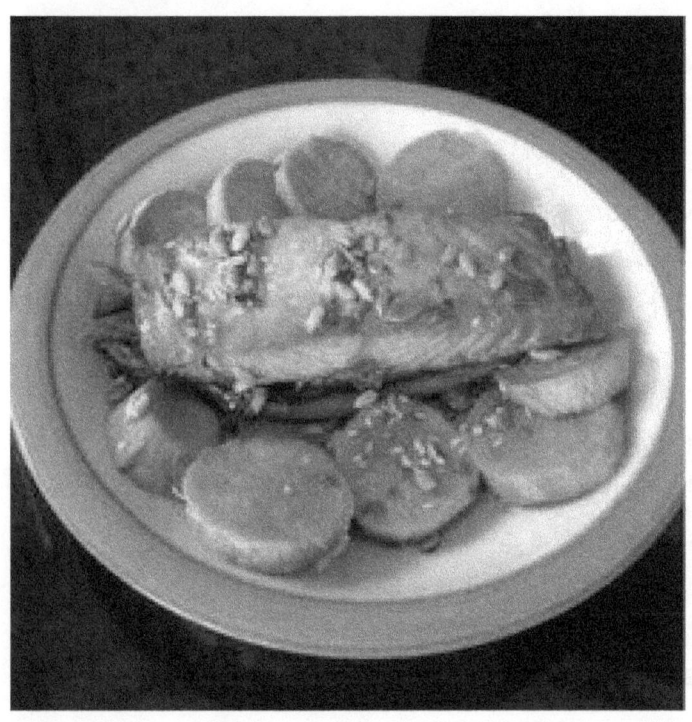

Ingredients

- 1/3 cup virgin olive oil
- ¼ cup each of coarsely chopped fresh oregano and fresh lemon juice
- 4 eight ounces salmon fillets
- 2 tablespoons vegetable oil
- 1 teaspoon minced garlic
- 1 lemon cut into quarters
- Sweet potato

Method

1. Preheat barbecue to medium heat. In a small bowl, mix olive oil, lemon juice, and oregano, and set it aside.

2. Gently rub vegetable oil and garlic into fillets, and season well. Grill for 4-6 minutes on each side.

3. Bring a pot of water to a boil, and drop in the sweet potato. Allow it to cook for 6-8 minutes until tender. Serve the salmon with the sweet potato.

Snacks: Low Fat Homemade Yogurt & Roasted Nuts

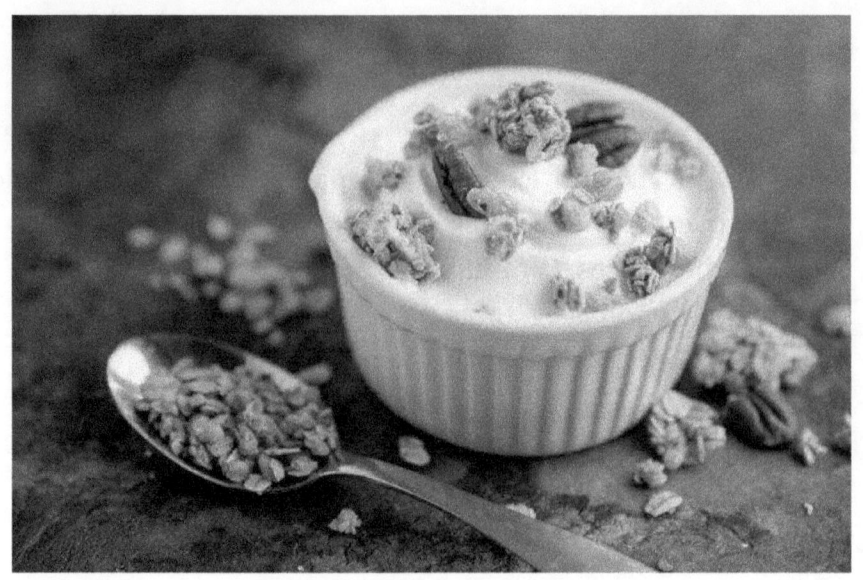

See Week 2 Day 1 For Yogurt Recipe

Week 2

Day 4

Breakfast: Boiled Oats with Butter & Homemade Yogurt

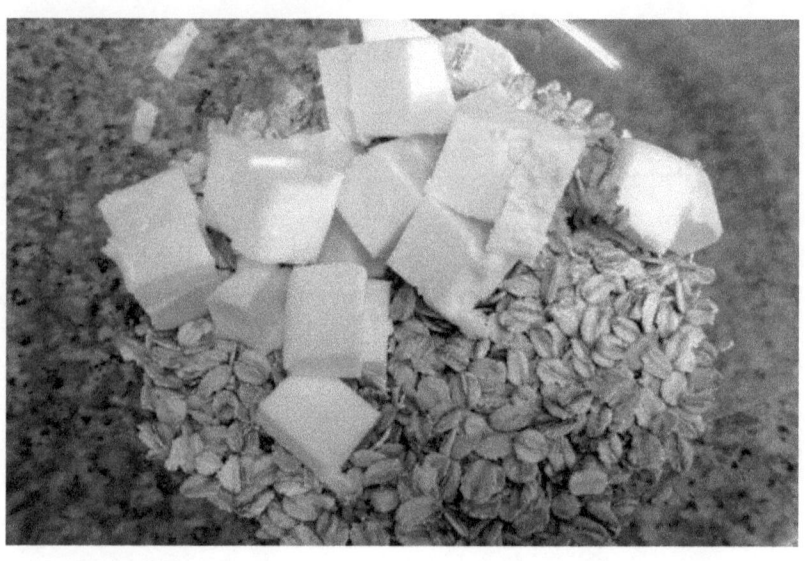

See Week 1 Day 4 For Boiled Oats Recipe

See Week 2 Day 1 For Yogurt Recipe

Lunch: Spicy Fried Chicken

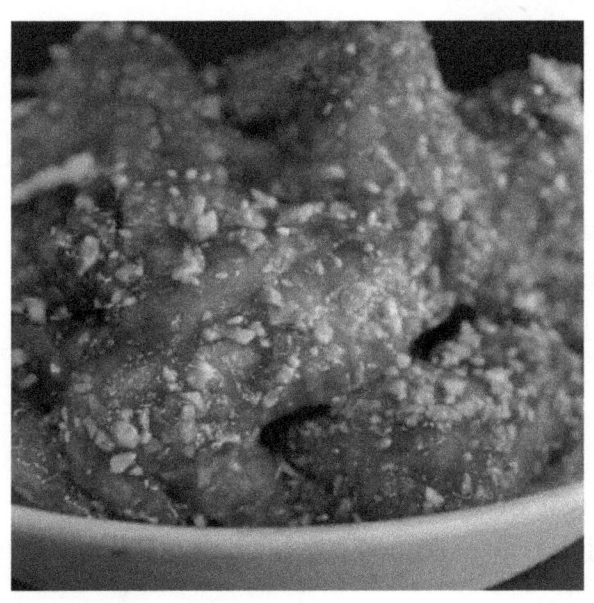

See Week 1 Day 1 For Recipe

Dinner: Potato & Pork Bake

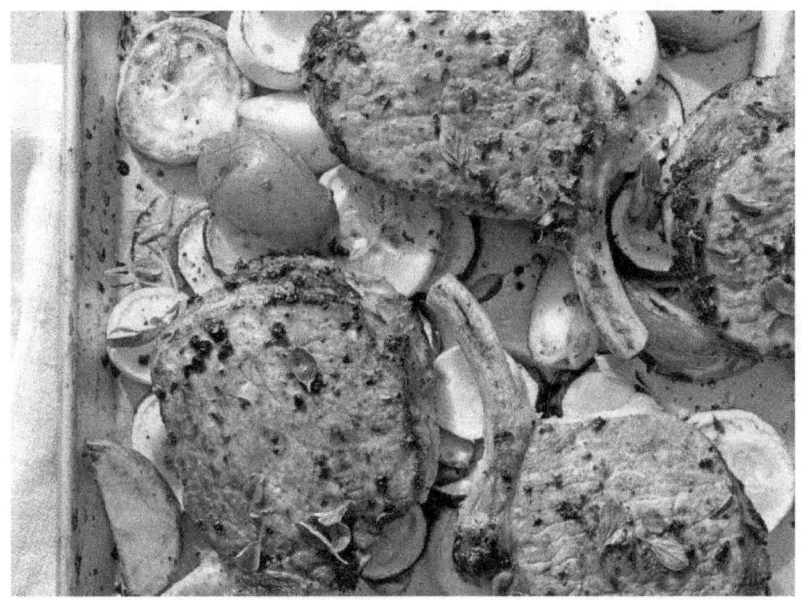

Ingredients

- 8 potatoes (cubed)
- 8 thick cut pork chops
- 1 onion (chopped)
- 1 tablespoon olive oil
- 1 cup vegetable stock

Method

1. Preheat oven to 200 degrees C. Place the potatoes in a baking tray. Arrange the pork chops over the potatoes.

2. Cook the onions in oil until they are slightly browned, and mix them with the stock.

3. Pour this mixture over the meat and potatoes. Bake for 30 to 40 minutes. Serve with a vegetable salad.

Snacks: Mixed Vegetable Smoothie & Fresh Fruit

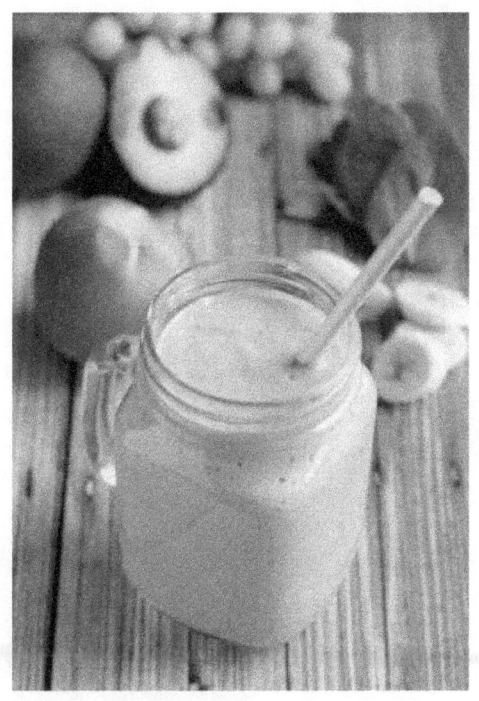

See Week 2 Day 2 For Smoothie Recipe

Week 2

Day 5

Breakfast: Egg & Potato Breakfast Casserole

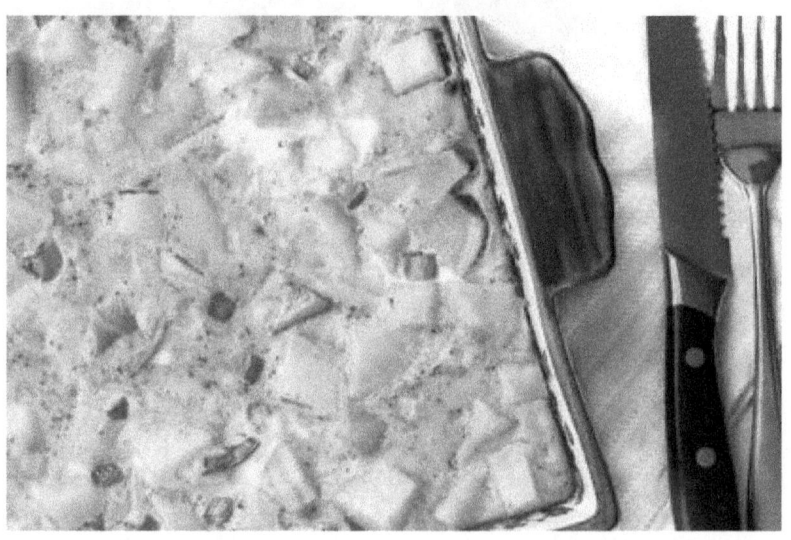

See Week 1 Day 1 For Recipe

Lunch: Taco Salad

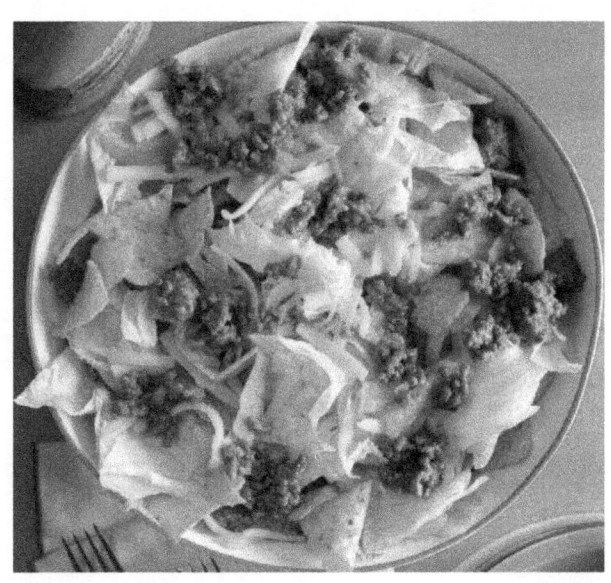

See Week 2 Day 3 For Recipe

Dinner: Macaroni & Cheese, Fruit Salad, & Steamed Cauliflower

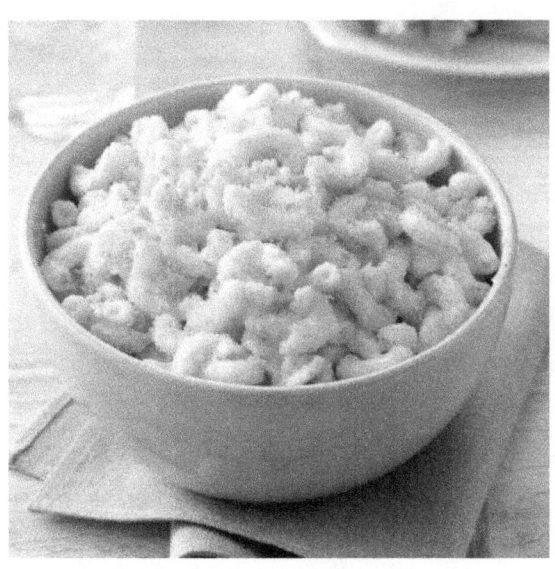

Ingredients

- 2 tablespoons extra virgin olive oil
- ¼ cup onion (chopped)
- 2 tablespoons flour
- 2 cups milk
- ¾ teaspoon salt
- ½ teaspoon dry mustard
- ¼ teaspoon pepper
- 8 ounces whole wheat macaroni
- 2 cups cottage cheese

Method

1. Preheat the oven to 175 degrees C. Heat a skillet over low heat, and add the olive oil.

2. Sauté the onions for 2 to 3 minutes until they become translucent. Stir in the flour. Cook for a minute or two, while stirring continuously.

3. Add the milk, salt, dry mustard, and pepper, and cook while stirring frequently to ensure lumps do not form. Remove the mixture from the heat after it boils, and allow it to thicken.

4. In the meantime, bring a pot of water to a boil. Add a pinch of salt and a capful of olive oil. Add the macaroni to the boiling water, and boil for 8 to 10 minutes. Macaroni is done when it sticks when thrown against a wall. Drain and cool the pasta.

5. Add the cheese to the milk mixture, and stir it in until it melts. Mix macaroni and the cheese sauce together, and place everything in a baking dish.

6. Bake for about thirty minutes or until bubbly and a little browned. Allow the macaroni to cool for about ten minutes, and then serve with fruit salad and steamed cauliflower.

Snacks: Dried Fruit & A Spinach & Broccoli Smoothie

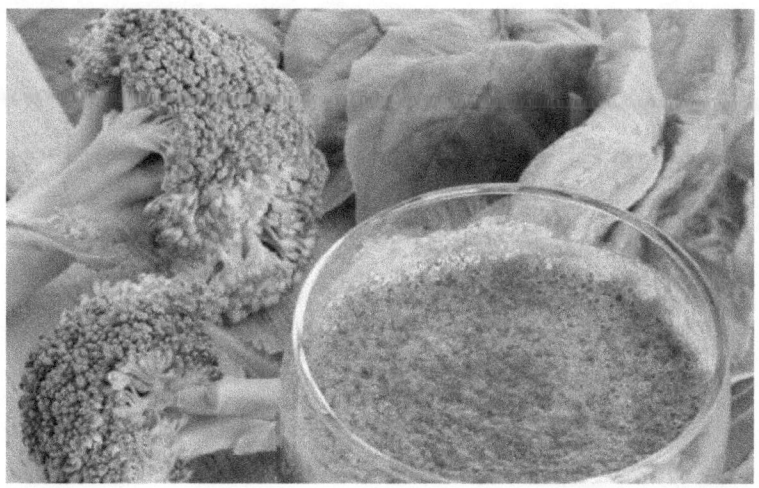

Ingredients

- 1 carrot
- 4 florets of broccoli
- 2 handfuls of spinach
- 1 apple
- 2 oranges

- Water (to dilute as needed)

Method

1. Combine all ingredients in the blender, and blend until they are smooth.

Week 2

Day 6

Breakfast: Whole Wheat Pumpkin Waffles

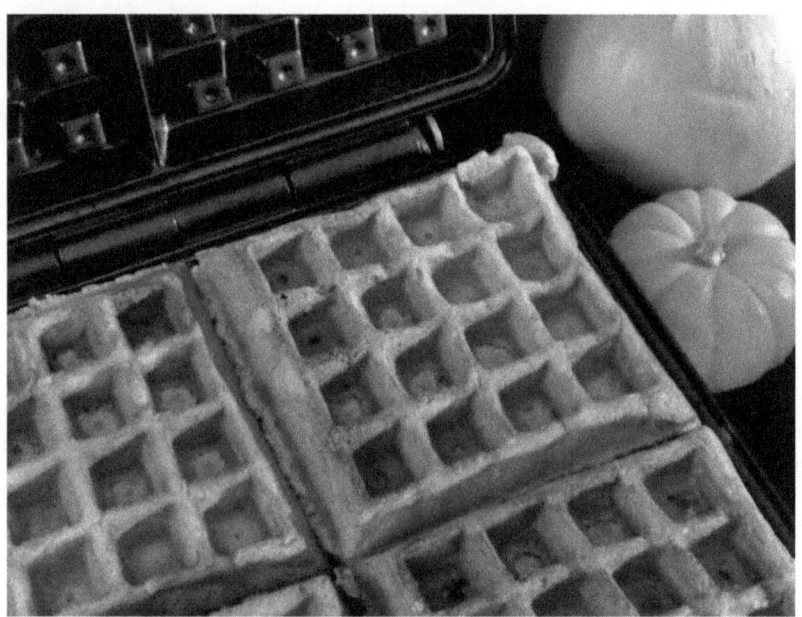

Ingredients

- 2 large eggs
- 2 tablespoons melted coconut oil
- 2 tablespoons pure maple syrup
- 1 teaspoon vanilla extract
- 1 cup plain low-fat yogurt
- ¾ cup pumpkin puree
- ½ cup low fat milk

- 1¼ cups whole wheat flour
- ½ cup ground flax seeds
- 1 tablespoon baking powder
- 1 tablespoon cinnamon
- 1 teaspoon nutmeg
- ½ teaspoon cloves
- ½ teaspoon salt
- Chopped walnuts
- Maple syrup (to top the waffles)

Method

1. Heat a waffle maker while you make the batter.

2. In a medium bowl, mix together the yogurt, pumpkin puree, milk, eggs, maple syrup, and vanilla extract.

3. In a different bowl, mix together the flour, flax seeds, baking powder, cinnamon, nutmeg, cloves, and salt.

4. Add the wet ingredients to the dry ingredients. Do this slowly so as not to over mix the batter.

5. Spoon the batter into the waffle maker in ½ cup intervals. Serve with walnuts and maple syrup.

Lunch: Tuna & Plain Yogurt Sandwich

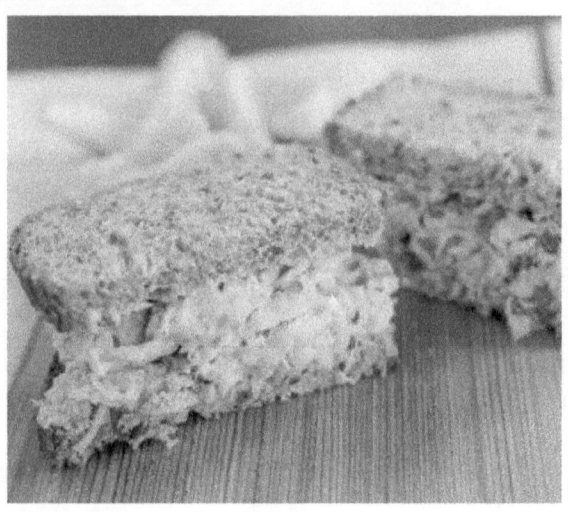

Ingredients

- 1 can of tuna
- 2 tablespoons onion (minced)
- 3 tablespoons dill pickles (finely chopped)
- 1 tablespoon dried parsley
- ¼ cup nonfat yogurt
- ½ teaspoon Dijon mustard
- ¼ teaspoon ground black pepper
- 2 pieces whole wheat bread

Method

1. Combine all ingredients, except the bread. Mix them well until they are fully blended.

2. Spread on the two pieces of bread, and enjoy your sandwich!

Dinner: Pork Kebabs with Chimichurri

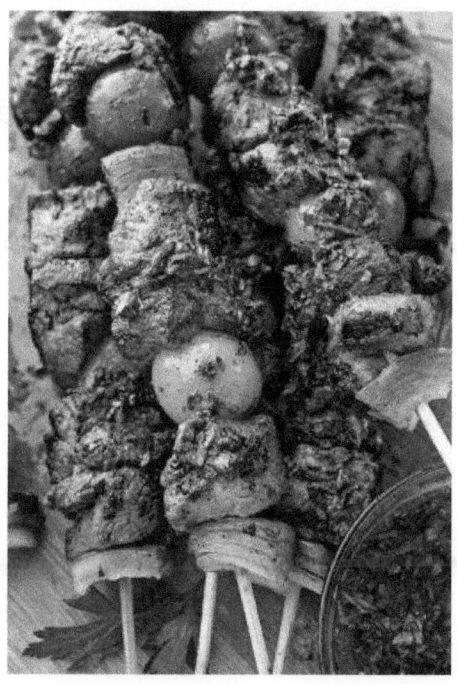

Ingredients

- 1½ pounds pork rashers without rind
- 6 baby onions (peeled and halved)
- 1 tablespoon mustard
- 3 tablespoons honey
- 1 teaspoon each of chopped parsley and dried Italian herbs
- 1 red onions (chopped)
- ½ cup olive oil
- 2 tablespoons lemon juice
- 2 garlic cloves (chopped)
- ½ teaspoon chili powder

- Salt and freshly ground pepper

Method

1. Preheat oven to 200 degrees C. Thread the meat and onions onto the kebob skewers.

2. Mix honey and mustard, and use the mixture to brush the kebabs. Arrange the kebabs on an oven rack, and bake for 12-15 minutes.

3. Mix all the chimichurri ingredients (everything remaining) while the kebabs bake. Serve kebabs with chimichurri and a salad.

Snacks: Mixed Fruit Smoothie & Roasted Nuts

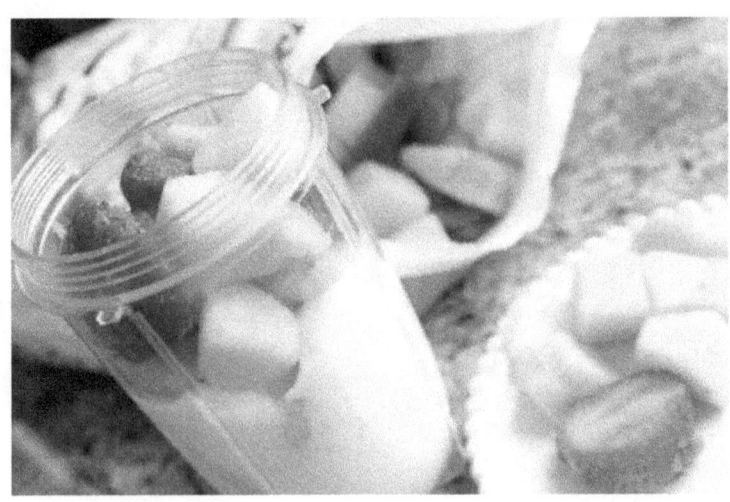

Week 2

Day 7

Breakfast: Steel Cut Oats

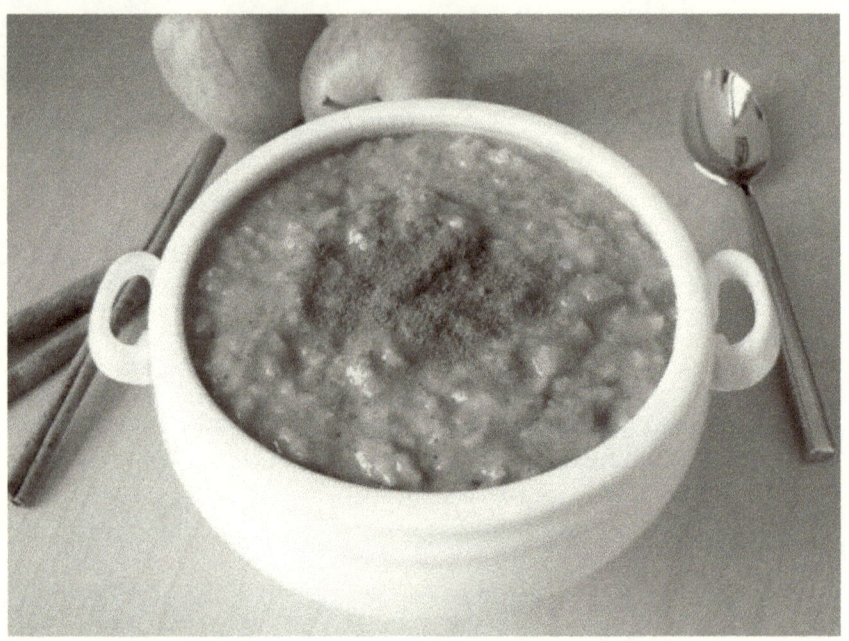

Ingredients

- ½ cup whole milk
- ½ cup plus 1 tablespoon low fat buttermilk
- 1 tablespoon brown sugar
- ¼ teaspoon cinnamon
- 1 tablespoon butter
- 1 cup steel cut oats
- 3 cups of water

Method

1. In a large pot, melt the butter. Add the oats, and stir for 2 minutes. Add the boiling water, and reduce the heat to a simmer. Cook for 25 minutes.

2. Combine the milk and half of the buttermilk with the oatmeal mixture. Stir everything gently to combine it, and cook for about 10 more minutes.

3. Once the oatmeal is finished cooking, spoon it into a bowl and top it with cinnamon, brown sugar, and remaining buttermilk.

Lunch: Grilled Chicken Wrap

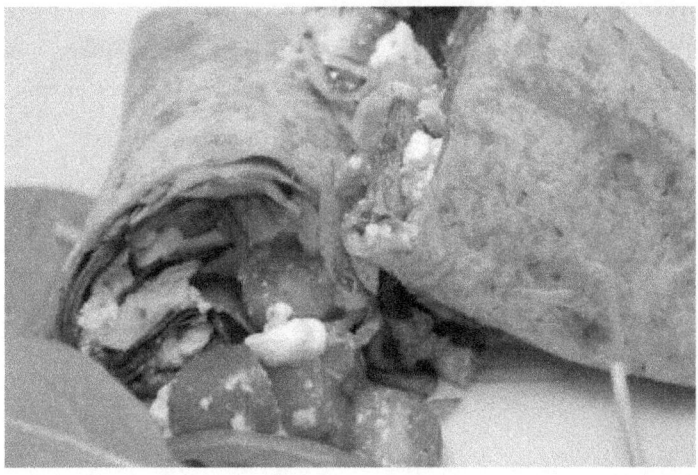

Ingredients

- 1-pound chicken (skinned, bones removed, cut into bite-sized pieces)

- 1/2 teaspoon pepper
- 3 tablespoons plain Greek yogurt
- 3 tablespoons apple cider vinegar
- 3 tablespoons onion
- 2 tablespoons extra-virgin olive oil
- 1/8 teaspoon salt
- 1 medium tomato
- 1 avocado
- 3 strips cooked bacon (optional)
- 8 large leaves red- or green-leaf lettuce
- 4 10-inch whole wheat tortillas

Method

1. Preheat a grill to medium-high heat. Sprinkle chicken with half of the pepper.

2. Spray the grill with a non-stick cooking spray, and grill the chicken, turning once or twice, for about 15 minutes. Remove from the heat, and let it cool for about 5-6 minutes.

3. While the chicken is cooking, mix together the onion, oil, vinegar, yogurt, salt, and the remaining pepper in a bowl.

4. Add the chicken, tomato, and avocado to the bowl. Lay out a tortilla. Add 2 lettuce leaves and a scoop of the chicken mixture. Wrap it up like a burrito, and enjoy!

Dinner: Grilled Salmon & Boiled Sweet Potato

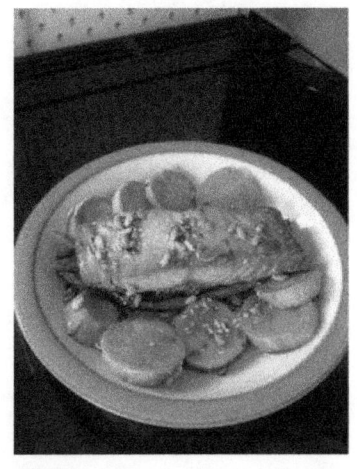

See Week 2 Day 3 For Recipe

Snacks: Pineapple Tidbits & String Cheese

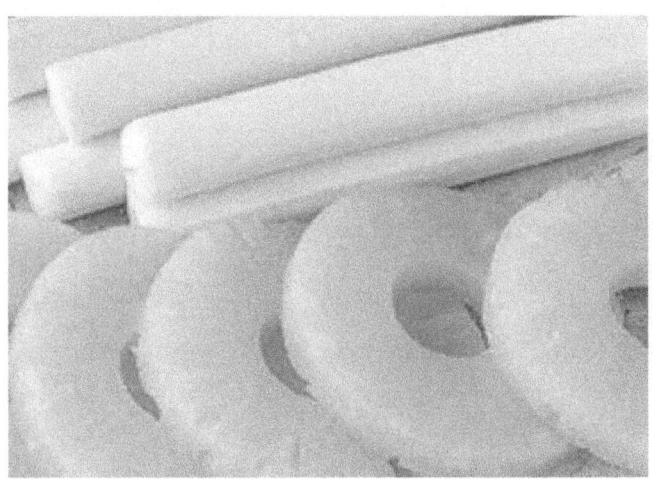

Once again, thank you for reading this book, and I hope you're getting a lot of valuable information. I would greatly appreciate it if you could take 30 seconds to leave me a review for this book on Amazon.com.

Week 3

Day 1

Breakfast: Banana Waffles

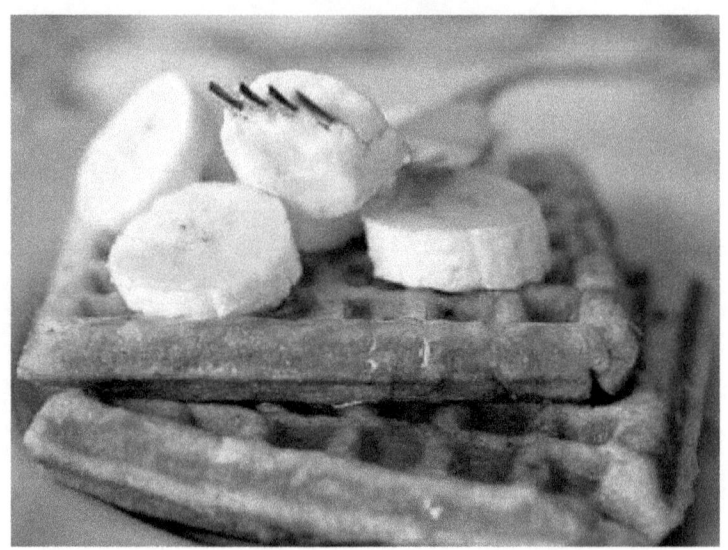

Ingredients

- 2 bananas
- 2 eggs
- ½ teaspoon vanilla extract
- ½ teaspoon baking powder
- ½ teaspoon ground cinnamon
- Pinch of salt
- ½ cup oats
- 1 tablespoon flour
- Chopped almonds

Method

1. In a bowl, mash up one banana with a fork. Add the eggs, vanilla extract, baking powder, cinnamon, and salt. Mix them all together.

2. Use a blender to blend the oats into a flour. Add the all-purpose flour to the oat flour, and mix it with the banana mixture.

3. Heat up the waffle iron, and pour in ½ cup of the batter. Bake for 2-3 minutes. Serve with a sliced-up banana and chopped almonds.

Lunch: Chicken & Avocado Sandwich

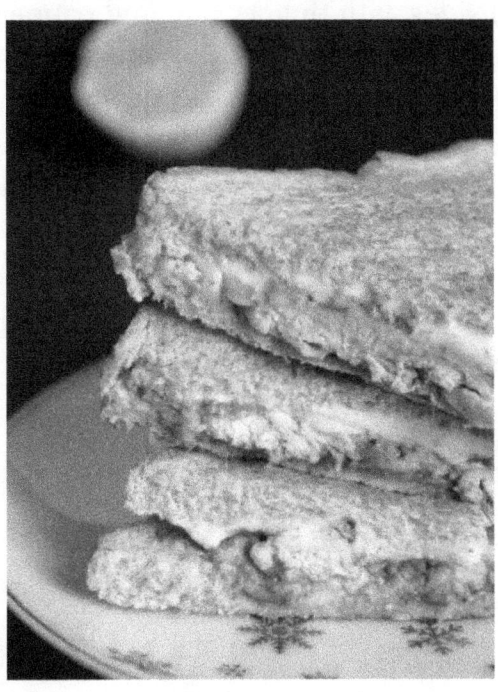

Ingredients

- 4-ounce chicken breast
- ¼ avocado
- 2 slices bread (preferably whole wheat)
- Romaine lettuce
- 1 teaspoon olive oil
- Pinch of thyme
- Pinch of pepper
- Pinch of salt
- 2 tablespoons low-fat mayonnaise

Method

1. Cut the chicken breast into strips. Season the chicken on both sides with thyme, salt, and pepper.

2. Heat the olive oil over medium-high heat. Once it is very hot, lay the chicken in the pan. Cook for 3-4 minutes on each side.

3. Toast the bread and cut up the avocado. Spread the mayonnaise on the bread. Build the sandwich with the finished chicken, avocado, and lettuce.

Dinner: Clean Eating Pork Chops

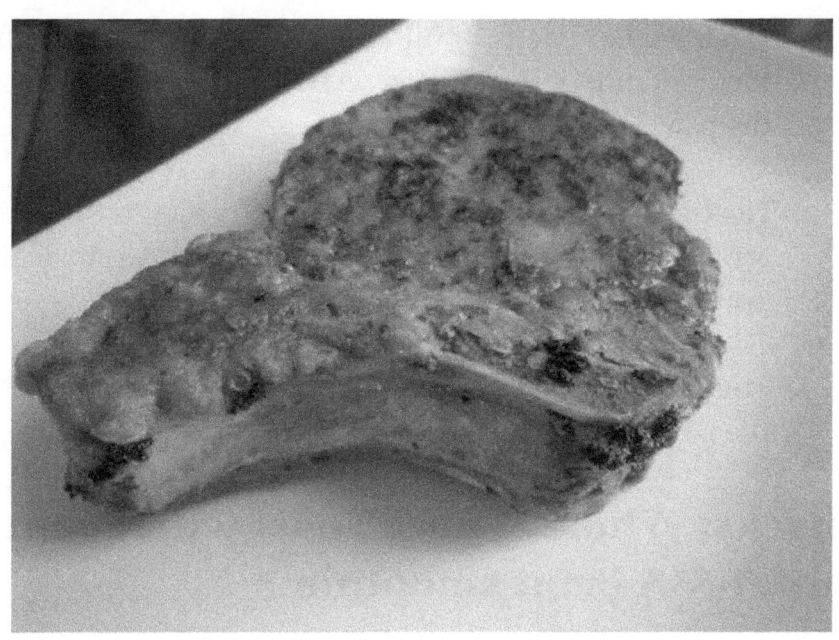

Ingredients

- 18 ounces pork chops
- 1 tablespoon flour
- 2 teaspoon dried rosemary
- 3 tablespoon olive oil
- 9 ounces sliced mushrooms
- Finely chopped garlic clove
- 1 1/3 cups vegetable stock

Method

1. Cut pork chops into finger thick strips. Coat well with a mixture of the rosemary, flour, and some salt and pepper.

2. Heat 2 tablespoons of oil in a wide frying pan, and fry the pork until it is browned on both sides. Remove from the pan.

3. Heat remaining oil in the pan, and fry the mushrooms for 2 minutes. Sprinkle in the garlic, and return the pork to the pan.

4. Stir in the stock until the mixture boils. Simmer until the pork is fully cooked. Serve with couscous or a salad.

Snacks: Whole Wheat Toast with Peanut Butter & A Fruit smoothie

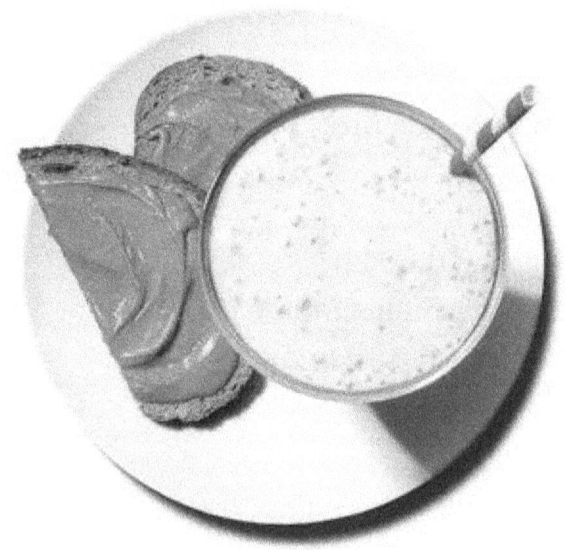

See Week 1 Day 1 For Smoothie Recipe

Week 3

Day 2

Breakfast: Raspberry Cinnamon Oatmeal & Eggs

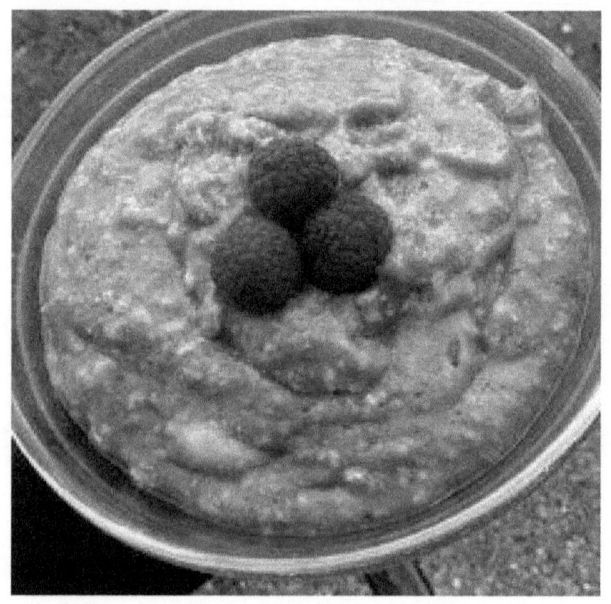

Ingredients

- 1/2 cup oatmeal (or oat bran)
- 1/2 cup milk of choice
- 1/2 cup water
- 1/2 tablespoon ground flax or chia seeds
- 3 egg whites
- 1 teaspoon cinnamon
- 1 packet Stevia

- 1 teaspoon vanilla
- 3/4 cup fresh raspberries
- 1 tablespoon nut butter (optional)

Method

1. Place all dry ingredients in a small pan. Add the milk, water, and vanilla. Turn on the heat, and allow it to simmer, stirring occasionally.

2. Add in the egg white and raspberries. Stir vigorously until the raspberries mix into the oatmeal and the eggs are fully cooked.

Lunch: Potato, Bacon, & Avocado Salad

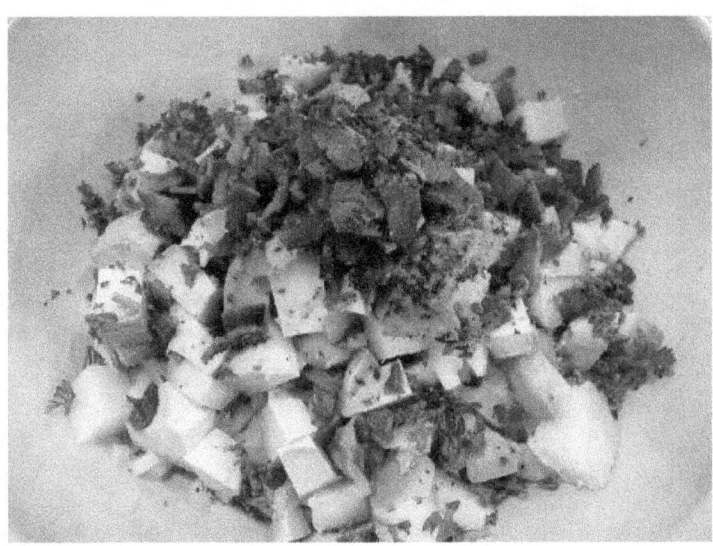

Ingredients

- 5 large red potatoes, scrubbed and cut into 1-inch chunks
- 6 ounces (or half a package) bacon
- 2 large avocados (mashed)
- 2 tablespoons sour cream
- 1 tablespoon lemon juice
- 1 teaspoon salt
- 1 teaspoon freshly ground black pepper
- 1 teaspoon garlic powder
- 1 teaspoon paprika
- 1 teaspoon red pepper flakes
- 2 tablespoons diced red onion
- 2 large eggs (hard-boiled and chopped)

Method

1. Boil potatoes until they are fork-tender, about 15-20 minutes. Drain and let them cool while you cut the bacon.

2. Slice the bacon into ½-inch strips, and cook in a non-stick skillet over medium-high heat until crispy, about 5-8 minutes. Transfer to a paper towel lined plate to drain. Reserve a few pieces of bacon for garnish.

3. In a large bowl, mash the avocados until it is mostly smooth with just a few lumps. Add the sour cream, lemon juice, salt, pepper, garlic powder, paprika, red pepper flakes, and red onion. Mix until combined.

4. Add the hard-boiled eggs, potatoes, and bacon to the bowl. Toss until coated. Cover and chill for at least 15 minutes before serving. Garnish with reserved bacon.

Dinner: Baked Potato, Fruit, & Vegetable Salad

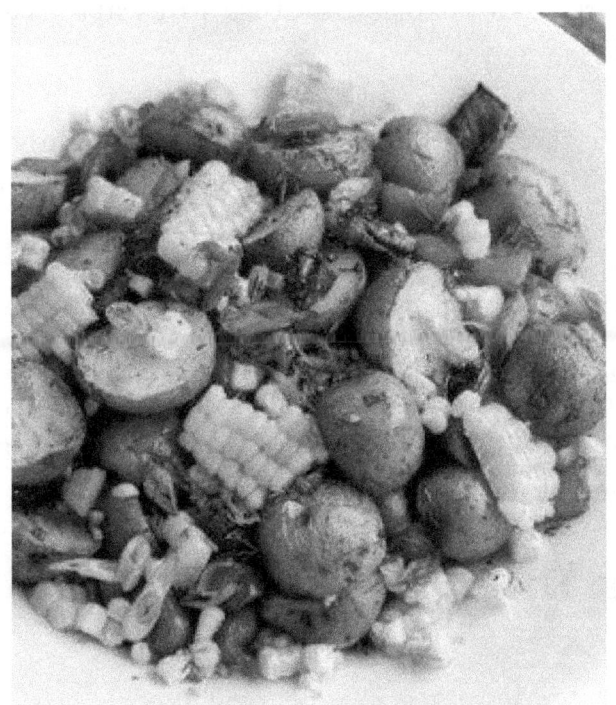

Ingredients

- 1 potato
- Olive oil
- Salt and pepper to taste

Method

1. Preheat oven to 170 degrees C. Thoroughly rinse the potato under cold running water, and wash it using a stiff brush.

2. Dry the potato, and then poke 10 to 12 deep holes using a fork; this enables moisture to escape as the potato cooks

3. Place the potato in a bowl and coat it lightly with olive oil.

4. Sprinkle all over with salt and pepper and place the potato on the middle oven rack.

5. Bake for about an hour or until the skin feels crisp and the inside feels soft. Serve with fresh fruit and a vegetable salad.

Snacks: Dried Fruits & Yogurt Smoothie

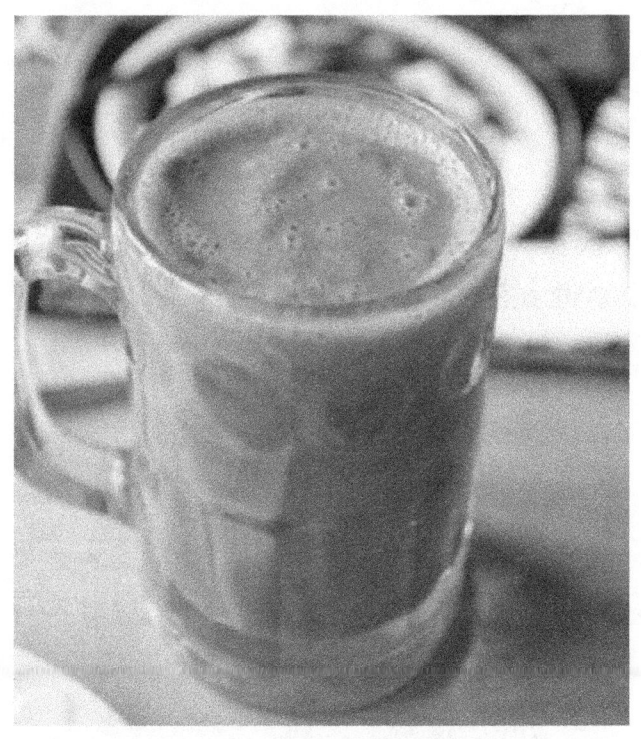

See Week 1 Day 1 For Recipe

Week 3

Day 3

Breakfast: Homemade Yogurt with Strawberries & Granola

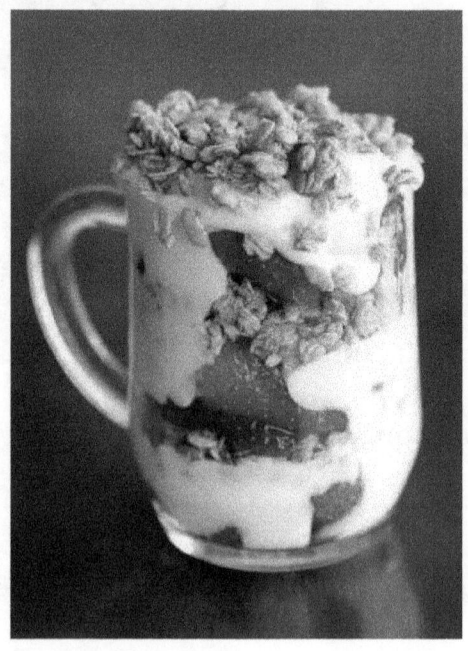

See Week 2 Day 1 For Recipe

Lunch: Mediterranean Tuna Salad

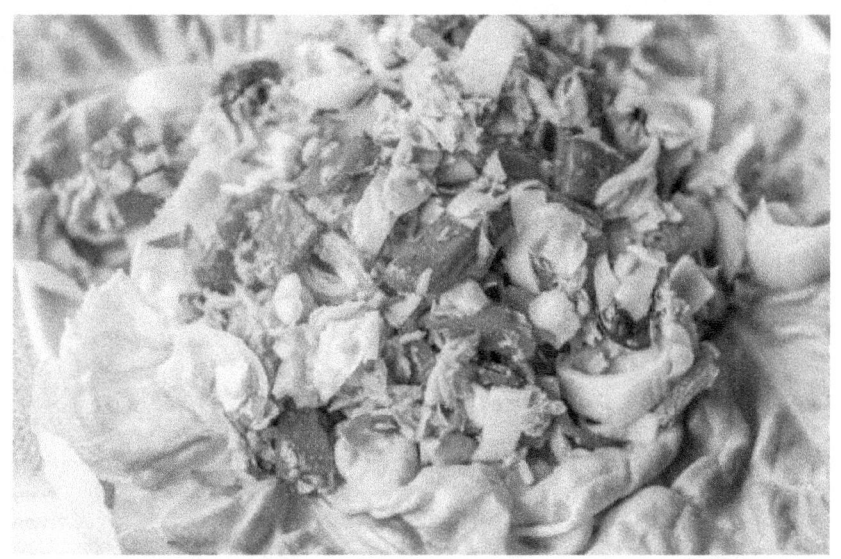

Ingredients

- 4 cans tuna (drained well)
- 1 can quartered artichoke hearts (drained)
- 1/2 cup chopped red bell peppers
- 3/4 cup sliced Greek olives
- 1/2 small red onion (finely chopped)
- 1/4 cup fresh flat-leaf parsley (chopped)
- 1/4 cup fresh basil (sliced)
- 2 cloves garlic (finely chopped)
- 1 teaspoon dried or 1 tablespoon chopped fresh oregano
- 1/2 cup mayonnaise
- 3 tablespoons lemon juice
- Salt and ground black pepper (to taste)

Method

1. Put all ingredients into a large bowl, and gently fold them together until well combined.

2. Serve on sliced bread as a sandwich or spoon over a green salad.

Dinner: Beef & Broccoli Stir Fry

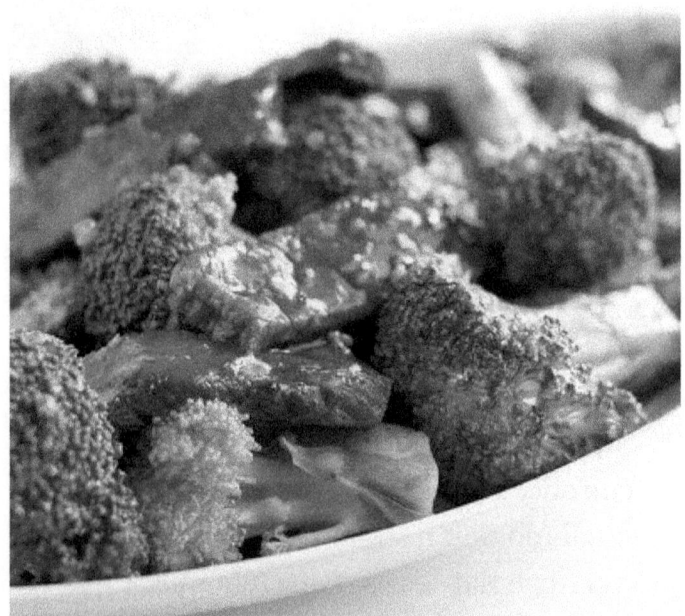

Ingredients

- 8 ounces sirloin steak
- 1 teaspoon cornstarch
- 2 tablespoons olive oil
- 1 onion (thinly sliced)
- 3 garlic cloves (minced)
- 1 tablespoon ginger (minced)
- 4 cups broccoli (chopped)

- ⅔ cup chicken stock
- ¼ cup hoisin sauce
- 2 tablespoons oyster sauce
- 2 tablespoons soy sauce
- 4 tablespoons cornstarch
- 1 tablespoon rice vinegar
- 1 teaspoon sesame oil
- ½ teaspoon chili paste

Method

1. Prepare sauce by whisking together all the sauce ingredients (hoisin sauce through chili paste). Set the sauce aside.

2. Cut beef into thin strips across the grain, and toss them with cornstarch. Heat 1 tablespoon of olive oil in a deep skillet over high heat.

3. Stir fry the beef for 3 minutes, and place it in a separate bowl. Add the remaining oil to the skillet, and stir-fry the onion, garlic, and ginger for a minute.

4. Add the broccoli and ½ cup of water, and steam for 3 minutes.

5. Pour in the sauce and stir together until the sauce thickens. Stir in beef and any juices for 3 minutes.

Snacks: Kale Apple Smoothie & Fresh Fruit

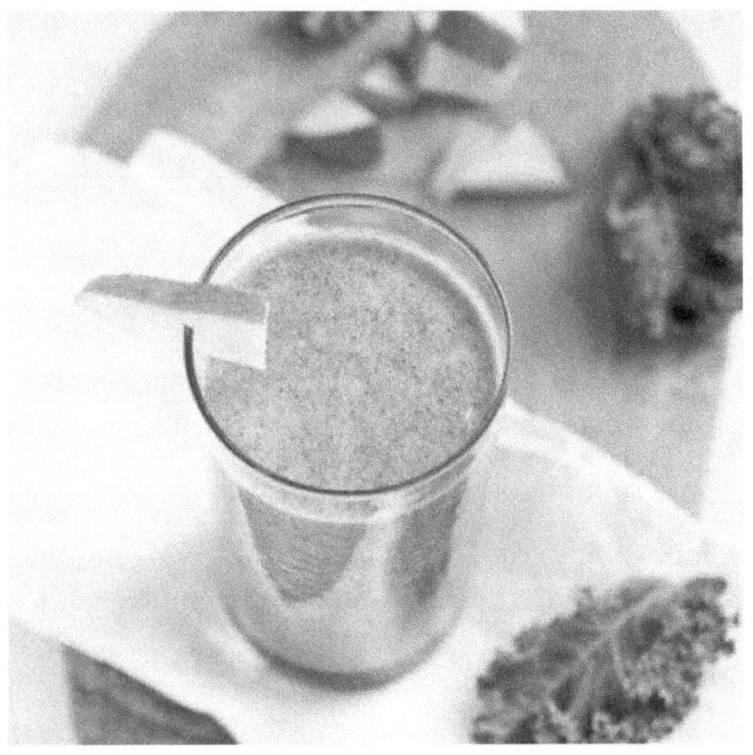

See Week 2 Day 2 For Recipe

Enjoying this book?

Check out my other best sellers!

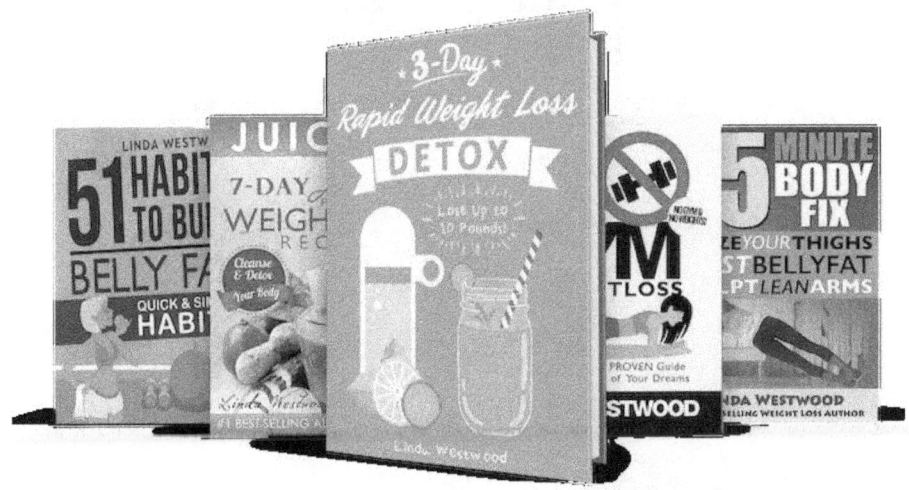

Get your next book on sale here:

TopFitnessAdvice.com/go/books

Week 3

Day 4

Breakfast: Waffles, Fresh Fruit, & An Egg

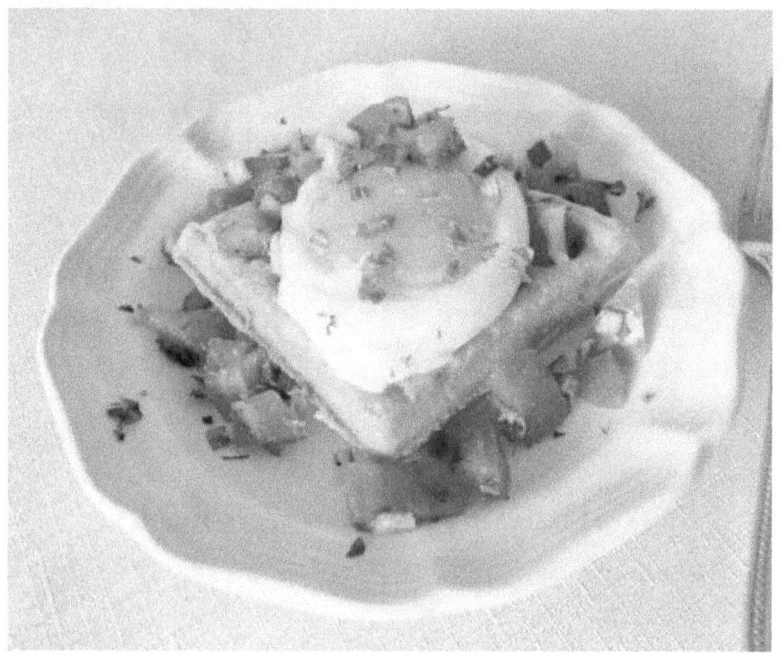

See Week 1 Day 7 For Waffle Recipe

Lunch: Chicken, Chickpea, & Tomato Salad

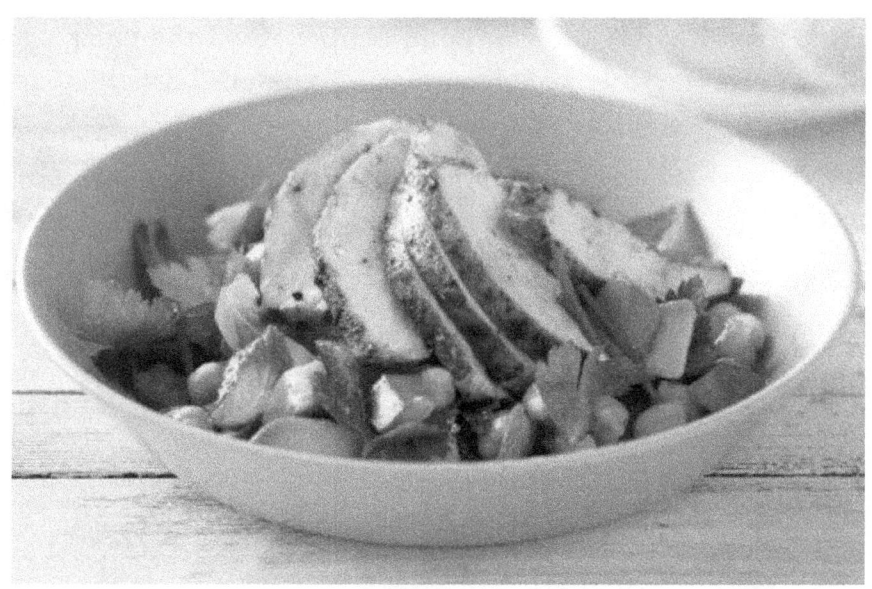

Ingredients

- ½ cup chickpeas
- 1 chicken breast (grilled however you would like)
- ½ cup tomatoes (chopped)
- 1 cup of arugula
- 1 teaspoon oregano
- 1 teaspoon salt
- ½ teaspoon pepper
- Fresh basil for garnish
- 1 tablespoon olive oil

Method

1. Rinse and dry the chickpeas thoroughly. Heat the oil in a pan over medium heat. Toss the chickpeas in the oil until they are warmed throughout.

2. Add the oregano, salt, and pepper. Coat the chickpeas. Combine the sliced chicken, tomatoes, arugula, and chickpeas. Top with the basil for garnish.

Dinner: Roast Sea Bass with Orange & Honey

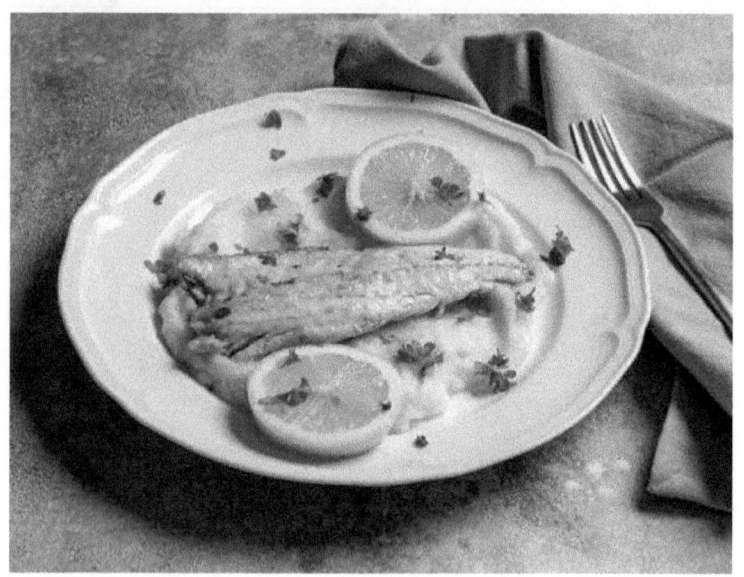

Ingredients

- 2 large sea-bass fillets
- Zest and juice ½ orange
- 2 teaspoon each honey and mustard
- 2 tablespoon olive oil
- 9 ounces ready-to-eat lentils
- 3 ounces watercress
- Small bunch each parsley and dill (chopped)

Method

1. Heat oven to 200 degrees C. Place the fillets skin-down on individual pieces of aluminum foil.

2. Mix the honey, zest, mustard, ½ oil, and some seasoning; drizzle mixture over the fillets. Pull the foil sides up, and twist the edges.

3. Place the foil "boats" on a baking tray, and bake for 10-12 minutes. Warm the lentils, and mix with the remaining ingredients.

4. Divide into 2 plates, place fish on top, drizzle on any leftover juices, and serve.

Snacks: Homemade Granola Cookies, & A Fruit Smoothie

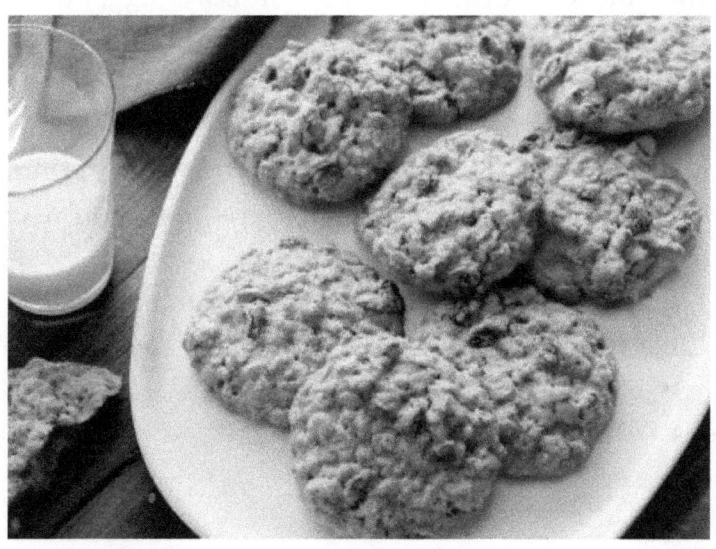

Ingredients

- 3 tablespoons butter (room temperature)
- ½ cup brown sugar
- ¼ cup honey
- 1 egg
- 1 tablespoon water
- ½ cup whole wheat flour
- ¼ teaspoon baking soda
- ½ teaspoon salt
- 1 ½ cups rolled oats

Method

1. Preheat oven to 175 degrees C. Spray a cookie sheet with nonstick cooking spray.

2. Using a mixer with the paddle attachment, mix together the butter, brown sugar, honey, egg, and water thoroughly.

3. Sift together the dry ingredients, and then stir in the oats. Add the dry ingredients to the wet and mix them together. Add any additional ingredients you've chosen.

4. Drop by heaping teaspoonfuls onto the cookie sheet. Bake 12 to 15 minutes. Cool on a wire rack.

See Week 1 Day 1 For Smoothie Recipe

Week 3

Day 5

Breakfast: Apple Cinnamon Slow Cooker Oatmeal

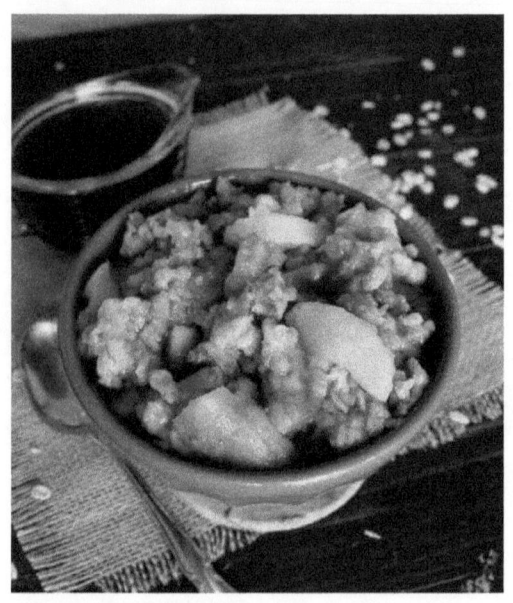

See Week 1 Day 2 For Recipe

Lunch: Overstuffed Vegetable Sandwich

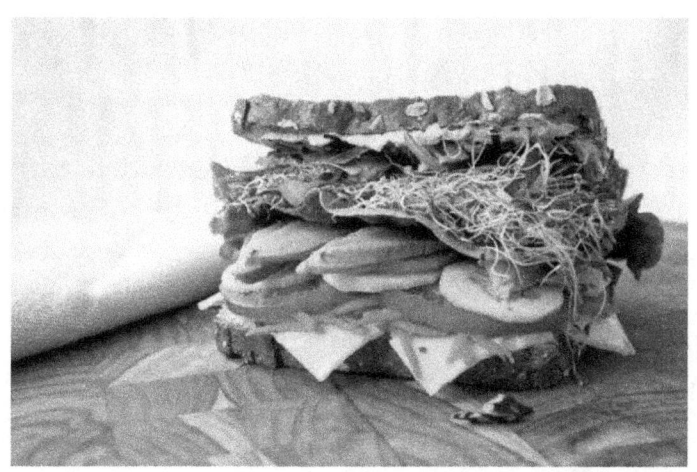

Ingredients

- 4 tablespoons Goat Cheese Yogurt Spread, goat cheese, Ranch Dip, or other creamy condiment of choice
- 8 slices whole grain/ whole wheat bread
- 4 large romaine lettuce leaves (or other lettuce) leaves, torn in half
- 1 medium sized avocado, peeled, pitted, and sliced
- 2 cups bean sprouts
- 1 large tomato (beefsteak works well), sliced
- 1/2 cucumber, peeled and sliced
- 1 cup grated carrots (peeled and grated on cheese grater)
- 4 slices low fat muenster, provolone, mozzarella cheese, or vegan cheese of choice
- Salt and pepper, to taste

Method

1. Spread 4 slices of bread with Goat Cheese Yogurt Spread or Ranch Dip Spread.

2. Add to the other slices cheese, shredded carrots, 1/4 cup bean sprouts to each, 2 slices of tomato, 1/4 avocado, and cucumber.

3. Top with the bread that has the spread on it then season with salt and pepper.

Dinner: Slow Cooker Jambalaya

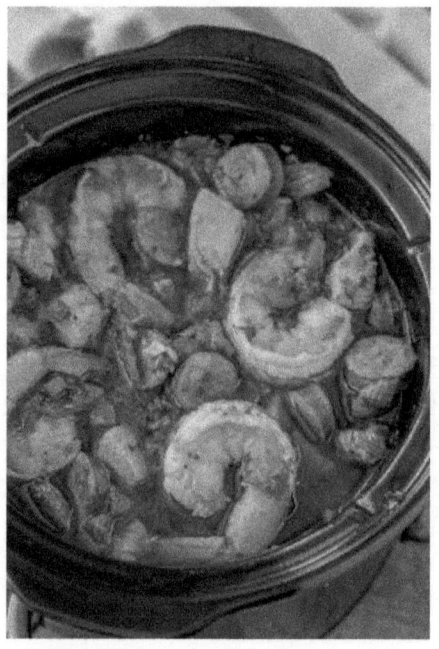

Ingredients

- 1 cup onion (chopped)
- 1 cup green pepper (chopped)

- 1 cup celery (chopped)
- 2 garlic cloves (minced)
- 1 28 ounces can undrained diced tomatoes
- ¾ pound cooked prawns
- 2 cups turkey sausage or smoked sausage
- ¼ teaspoon each of hot sauce and pepper
- ½ teaspoon each of salt and dried thyme
- 1 tablespoon dried parsley

Method

1. Add all ingredients, except prawns, to a slow cooker, and stir well.

2. Cook on high heat for 3-4 hours. Add prawns for the last 15 minutes of cooking time.

Snacks: Air-Popped Popcorn & Roasted Nuts

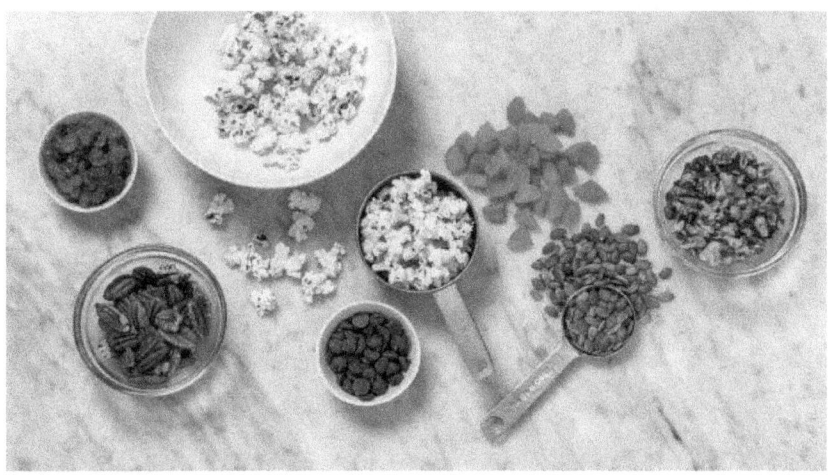

If you're enjoying this book and would love to let other potential readers know how great it is, please take a few seconds to leave a review on Amazon.com.

Week 3

Day 6

Breakfast: Boiled Oats with Dried Fruit

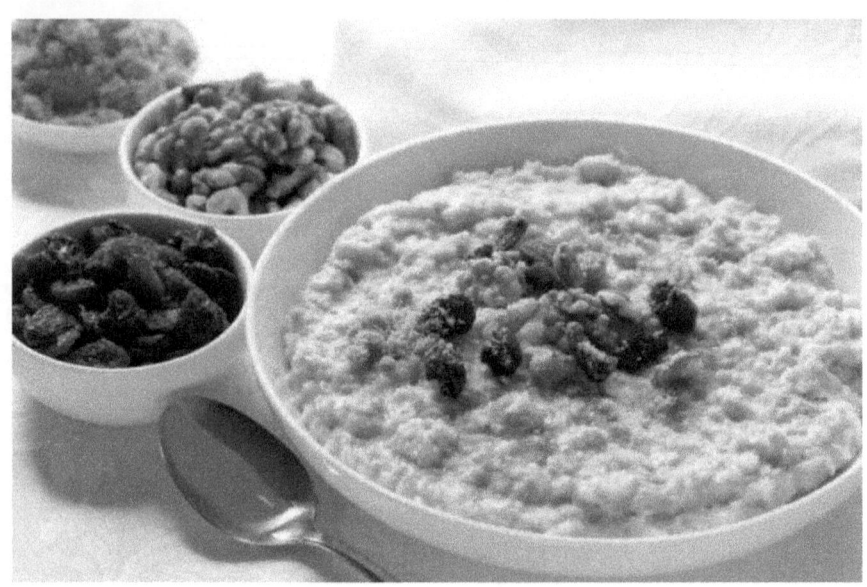

See Week 1 Day 4 For Recipe

Lunch: Chicken & Avocado Sandwich

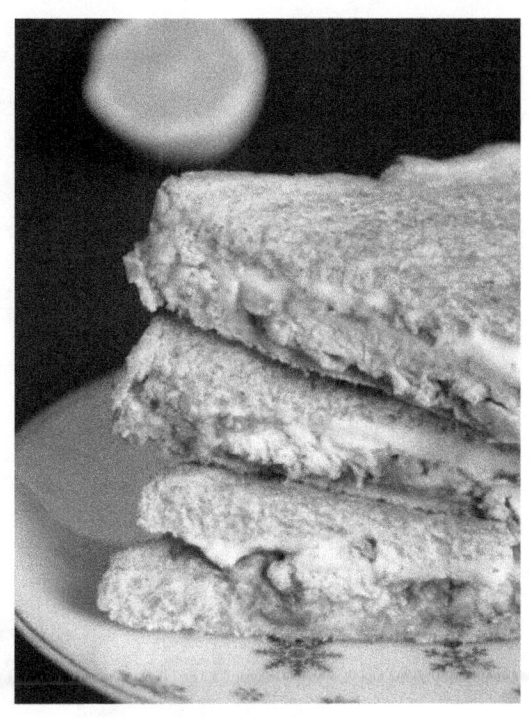

See Week 3 Day 1 For Recipe

Dinner: Four Bean Salad, Meat Loaf, & Mashed Butternuts

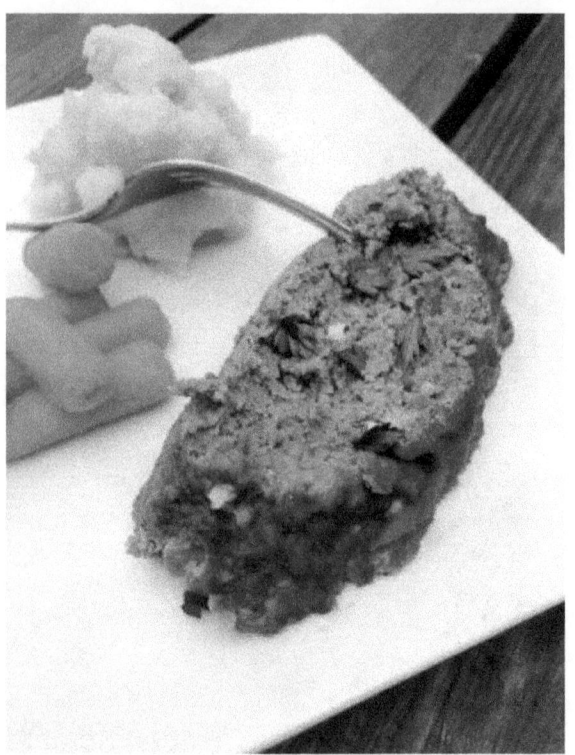

Ingredients

- 3 cups blanched green beans
- 2 cups cooked speckled red beans
- 2 ½ cups cooked white beans
- 2 each of green peppers and medium onions (sliced)
- 1 cup each white vinegar and olive oil
- 3 tablespoons caster sugar
- ½ cup chopped fresh coriander
- Salt and pepper

Method

1. Place beans, peppers, and onions into a salad bowl, and mix gently.

2. Put the remaining ingredients into a jug, and whisk briskly to make the salad dressing.

3. Sprinkle the salad dressing over the salad, and immediately serve with meatloaf and mashed butternut

Snacks: Air Popped Popcorn & Fresh Fruit

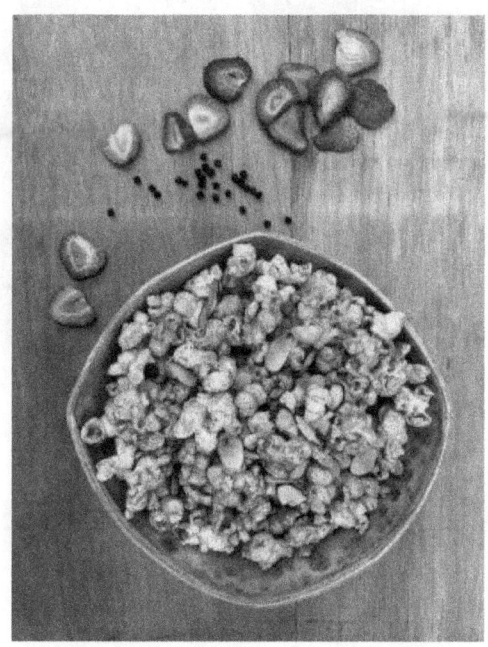

Week 3

Day 7

Breakfast: Tofu Scramble

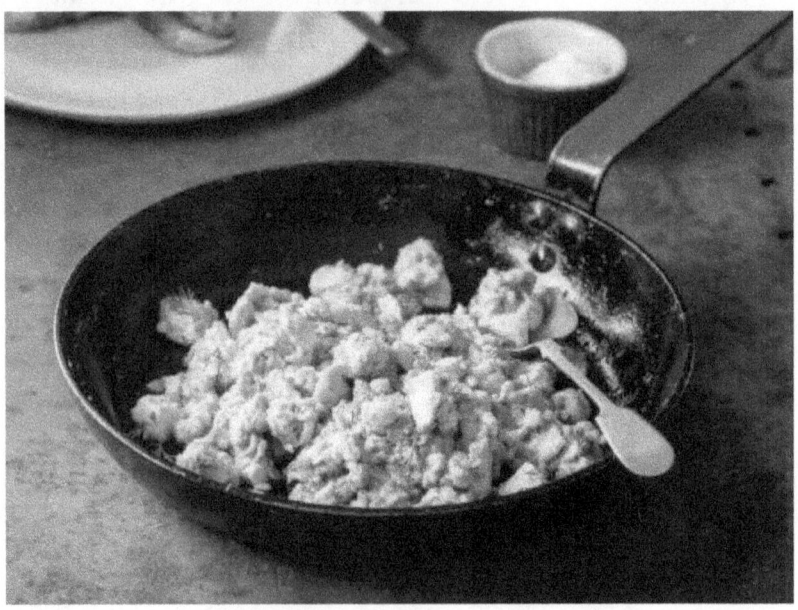

See Week 1 Day 5 For Recipe

Lunch: Asian Chicken Sandwich

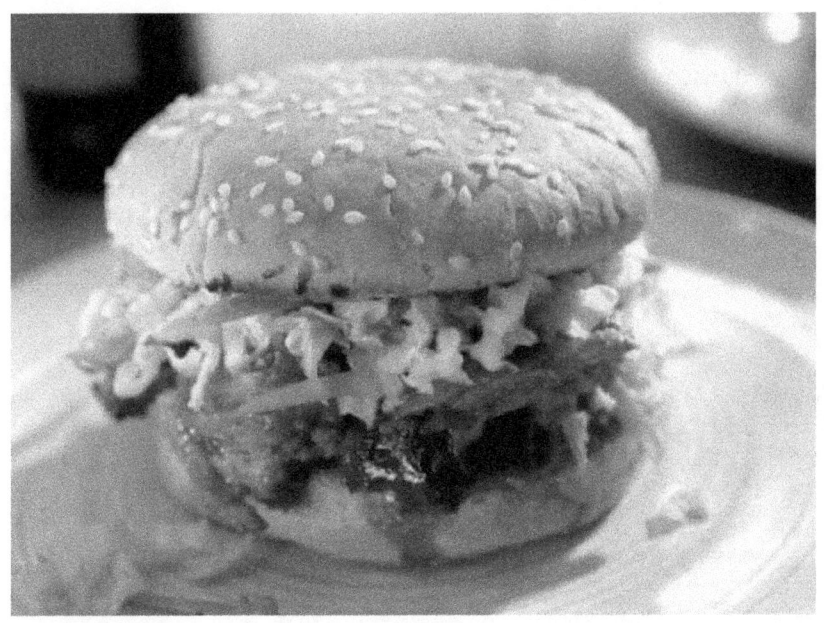

Ingredients

- 1 pre-cooked rotisserie chicken
- 1/2 cup light mayonnaise
- 2 teaspoons sesame oil
- 1 tablespoon sesame seeds
- 2 scallions
- 1/2 red bell pepper
- 4 rolls
- Salt
- Pepper

Method

1. Remove the meat from the chicken, chop it up into bite-sized pieces, and put it in a large bowl.

2. Add the mayonnaise, sesame oil, sesame seeds, scallions, and red pepper, salt, and pepper. Divide the mixture evenly between the four rolls. Enjoy!

Dinner: Spiced Salmon with Chili Sauce

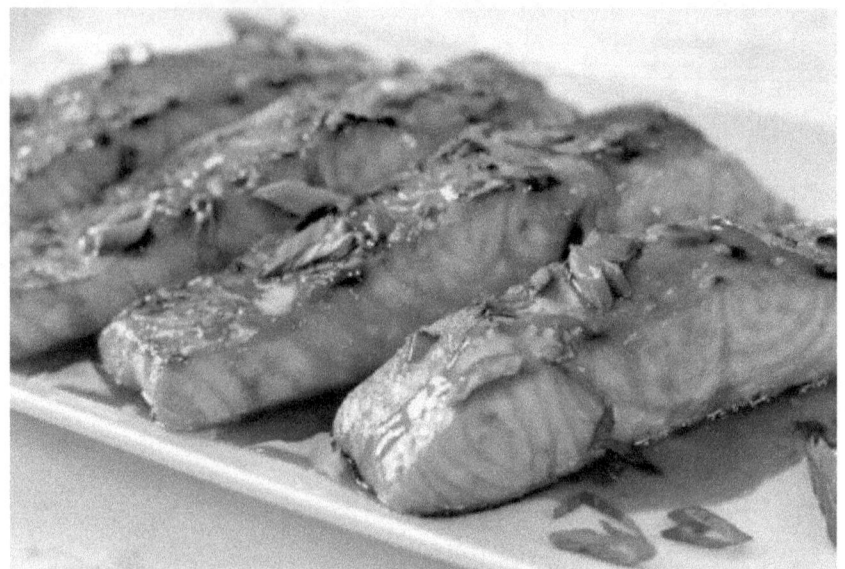

Ingredients

- 4 skinless salmon steaks
- ½ cup spicy Thai sauce
- 2 tablespoon soy sauce
- 2 tablespoons orange juice

Method

1. Preheat oven to 205 degrees C. Grease an ovenproof dish with cooking spray, and place fish inside the dish.

2. Mix the sauces with the orange juice, and pour over the fish fillets. Bake for 15 minutes. Serve with couscous.

Snacks: Veggies with Hummus & Fresh Fruit

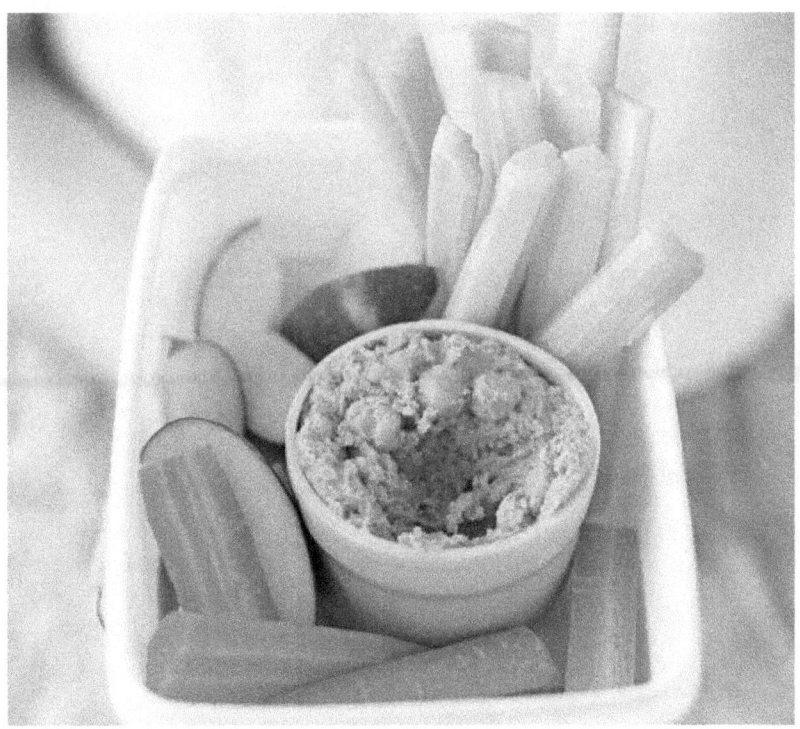

Week 4

Day 1

Breakfast: Turkey & Spinach Frittata

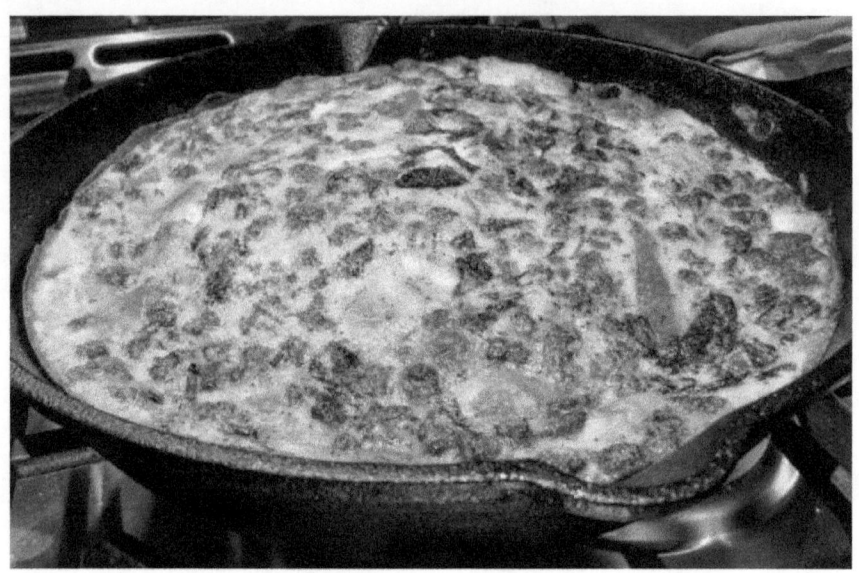

Ingredients

- 1 small onion
- 1/2 medium green pepper
- 1 garlic clove
- 1 Tablespoon vegetable oil (canola oil is also fine)
- 1 cup chopped spinach
- 1 cup cooked turkey
- 6 large eggs
- 1/4 cup heavy cream
- 1/4 teaspoon salt

- 1/4 teaspoon pepper

Method

1. Preheat the oven to a broil. Heat the oil in a large skillet on medium heat. Toss in the onion, green pepper, and garlic. Cook for 3-4 minute until they begin to look translucent.

2. Reduce the heat to medium low. Stir in the spinach and cook for about 2 more minutes. Add the turkey.

3. Meanwhile, mix together the eggs, cream, salt, and pepper in a medium bowl.

4. Add the egg mixture to the skillet. Don't stir. Allow the mixture to cook about 5 minutes until the eggs begin to cook.

5. Move the skillet to the oven, and broil the 2-5 minutes until the eggs are fully cooked. Cut into pie shaped wedges.

Lunch: Spicy Fried Chicken

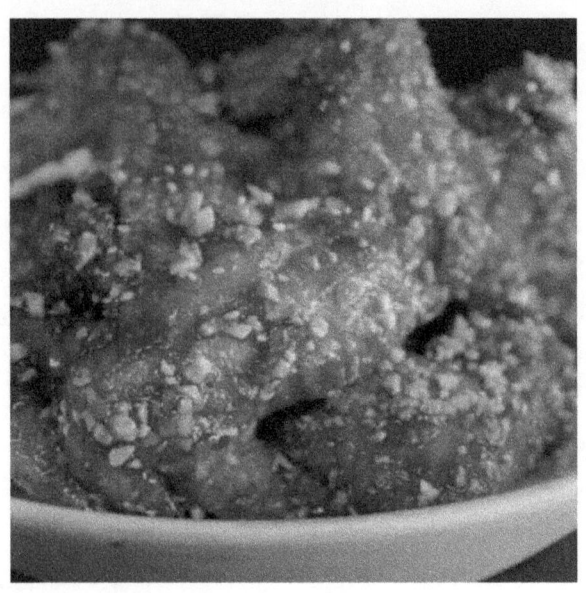

See Week 1 Day 1 For Recipe

Dinner: Mushroom & Cabbage Stroganoff

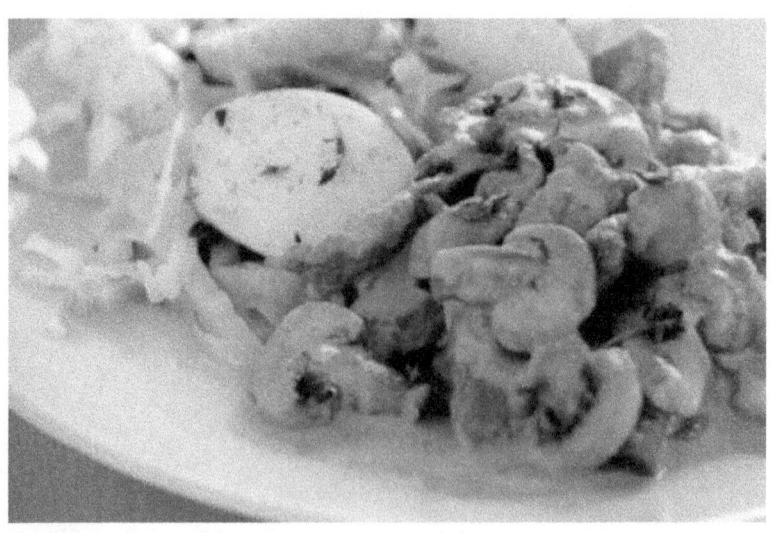

Ingredients

- 4 tablespoons oil
- 1 large onion (chopped)
- 2 tablespoons paprika
- 4 pounds mushrooms (sliced)
- 1 white and 1 red cabbages (shredded)
- 3½ cups vegetable stock
- 1-pound double cream
- Salt and pepper

Method

1. Heat oil in a large frying pan. Add the onions and fry until they are soft.

2. Add paprika, cabbage, and mushrooms and cook for 3 minutes. Add the stock. Simmer, covered, for about 8 minutes.

3. Add the cream and season well. Cook for a further 4 minutes before serving

Snacks: Raw Vegetable & Fresh Fruit

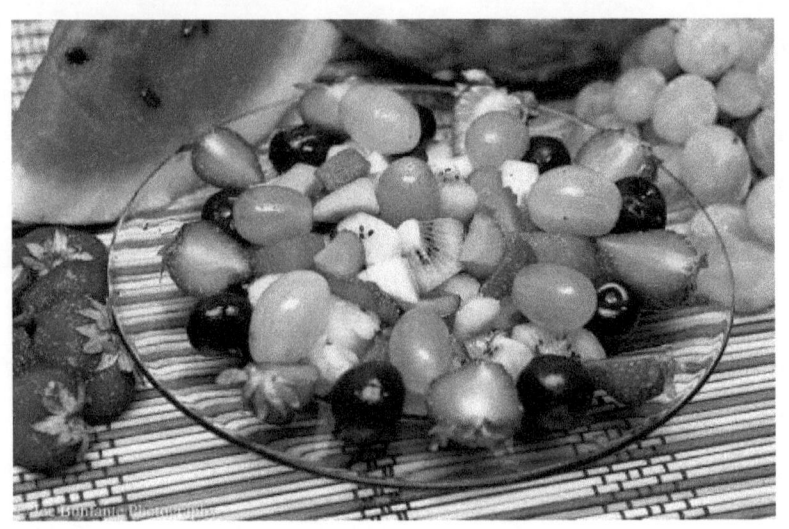

Week 4

Day 2

Breakfast: Homemade Yogurt, Eggs, & Toast

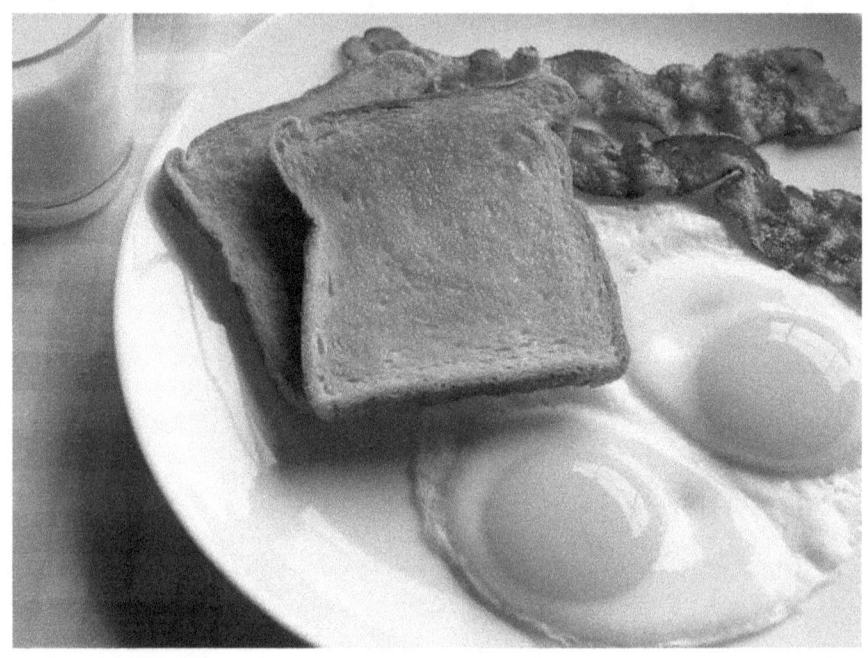

See Week 2 Day 1 For Recipe

Lunch: Chicken & Avocado Sandwich

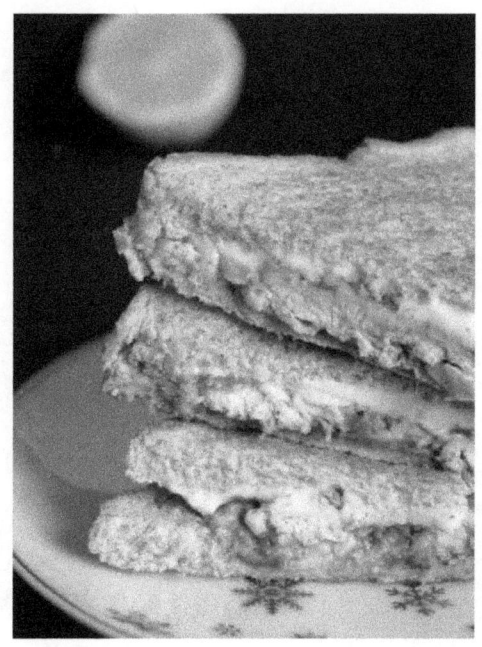

See Week 3 Day 1 For Recipe

Dinner: Fish & Baby Tomato Bake

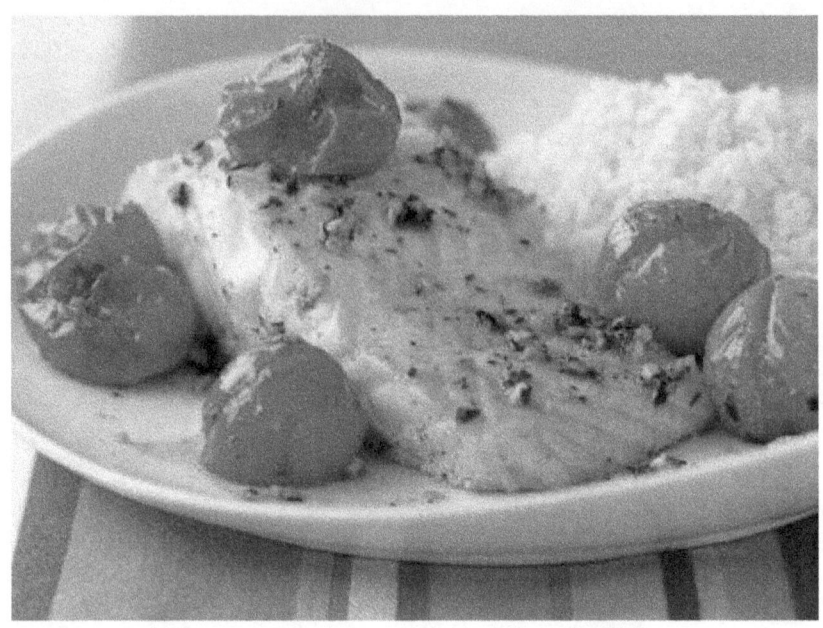

Ingredients

- 4-6 fish cutlets
- 1 tablespoon garlic and herb seasoning
- 4 ounces each of mixed baby tomatoes and steamed brussel sprouts
- Garlic bulb, halved horizontally
- 3 tablespoons olive oil
- Salt and freshly ground pepper

Method

1. Preheat oven to 200 degrees C. Grease an ovenproof dish with cooking spray.

2. Season the fish with garlic and herb seasoning, and place in the dish together with the tomatoes, garlic, and sprouts.

3. Drizzle with olive oil, and season with salt and pepper. Bake for 15 minutes. Serve with a salad.

Snacks: String Cheese & Fresh Fruit

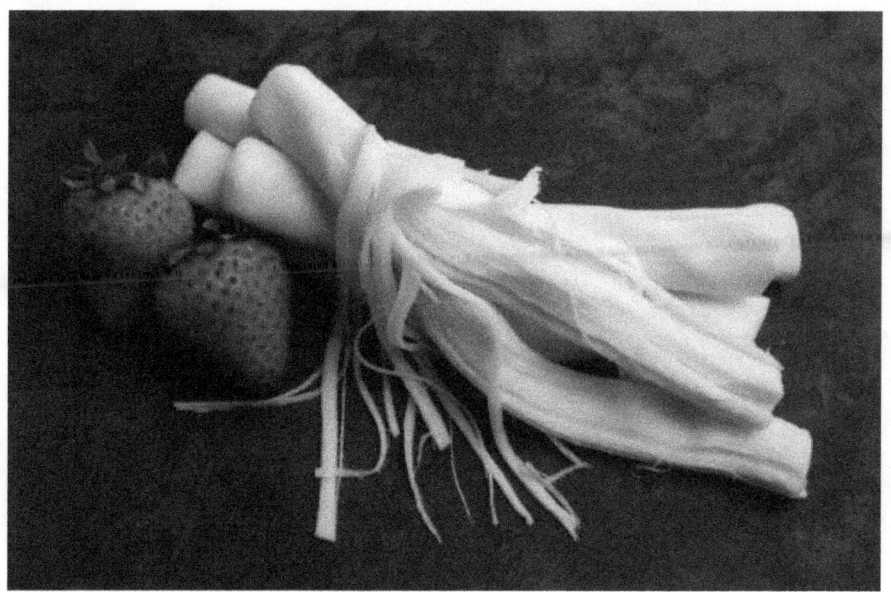

Week 4

Day 3

Breakfast: Carrot Cake Pancakes

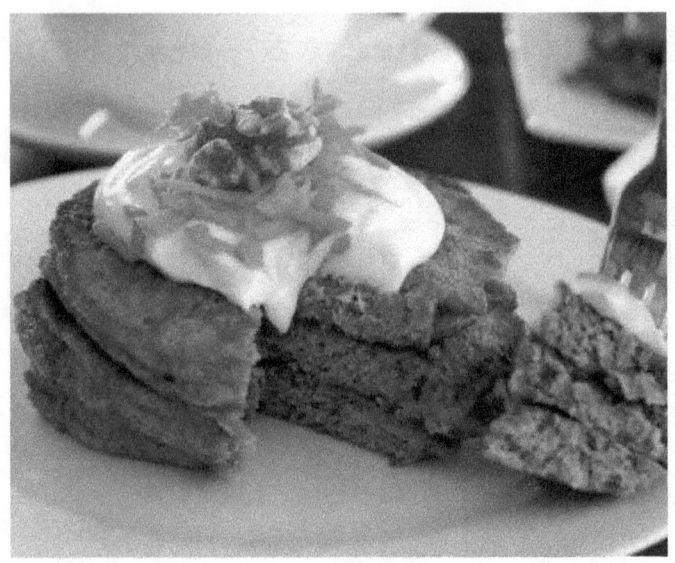

Ingredients

- 1 cup whole wheat flour
- 1 egg
- 2 tablespoons brown sugar
- 1 cup buttermilk
- 1 teaspoon vanilla extract
- 2 cups finely grated carrots
- 1 teaspoon baking powder
- ½ teaspoon baking soda
- ½ teaspoon salt

- ¾ teaspoon cinnamon
- ¼ teaspoon nutmeg
- ¼ teaspoon ginger
- Butter

Method

1. Put the cream cheese in a bowl, and set it aside until it reaches room temperature. Whisk together the baking soda, salt, flour, baking powder, nutmeg, ginger, and cinnamon.

2. In a different bowl, mix together the egg, vanilla, buttermilk, and brown sugar. Add the carrots to the dry mixture.

3. Add the wet ingredients to the dry ingredients. Stir everything together to incorporate, but do not over-stir.

4. On a hot griddle, heat up the butter, and then spoon the mixture into dollops to make the pancakes.

5. Serve them warm with butter, powdered sugar, syrup, or on their own.

Lunch: Overstuffed Vegetable Sandwich

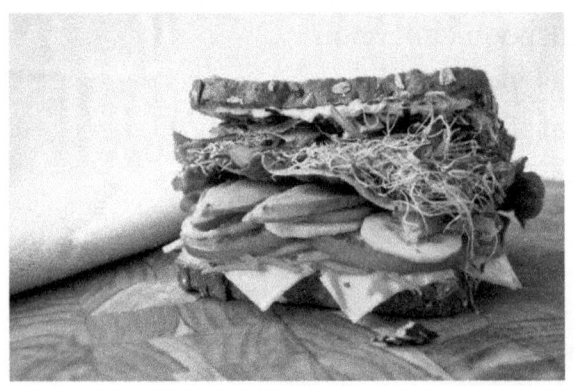

See Week 3 Day 5 For Recipe

Dinner: Slow Cooked Mexican Chicken

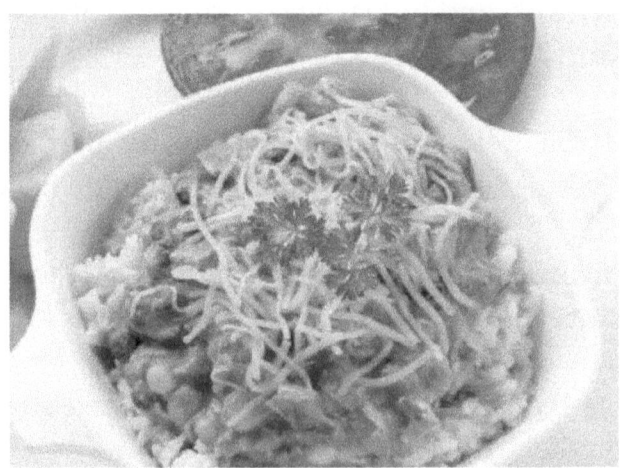

Ingredients

- 8 ounces chicken breasts
- 2 teaspoons taco seasoning
- ½ cup salsa
- 1 cup grated medium/ low fat cheddar cheese

Method

1. Spray the base and the sides of the slow cooker with cooking spray.

2. Season the chicken generously with taco seasoning on both sides, and spoon the salsa on top. Place in the slow cooker, and cook on low for 5-6 hours.

3. Open the lid, and sprinkle cheese evenly on the chicken breasts. Close the lid, and cook for a further 15 minutes.

Snacks: Yogurt & Spinach Smoothie & Air-Popped Popcorn

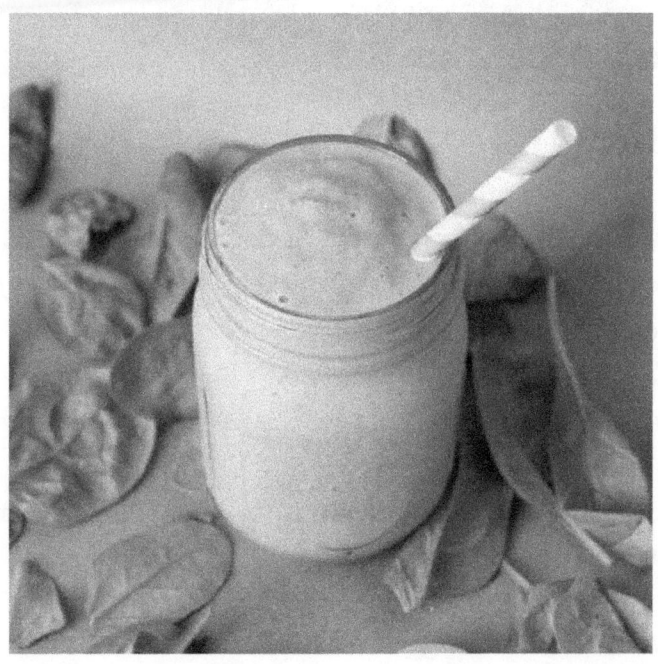

Week 4

Day 4

Breakfast: Whole Grain Cereal & Scrambled Egg

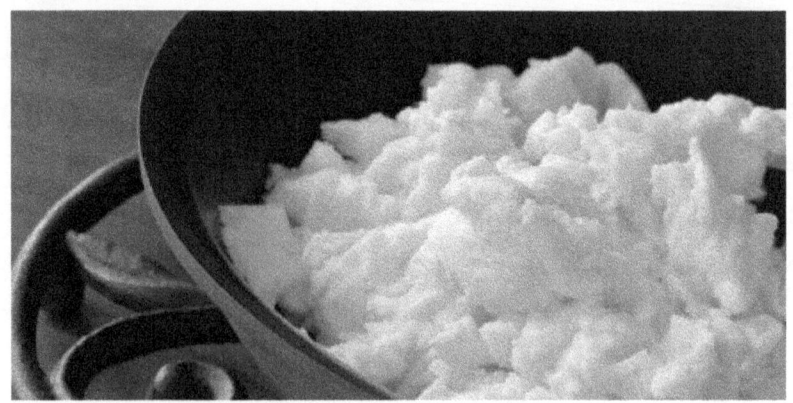

Ingredients

- ½ cup whole grain cereal of choice
- ¼ cup nonfat milk (or non-dairy milk of choice)
- 1 egg

Method

1. Scramble the egg over medium heat. Pour the milk over the cereal.

Lunch: Pork Carnitas With A Fruit Salad

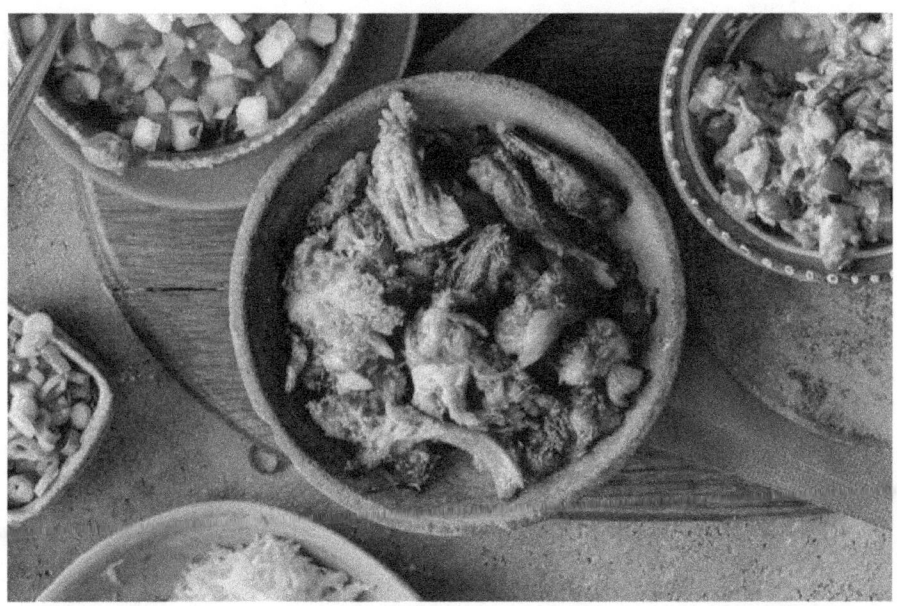

Ingredients

- 3 lb. pork roast
- 2 teaspoons salt
- 4 teaspoons chili powder
- 2 teaspoons cumin
- 1 teaspoon garlic powder
- 1 teaspoon black pepper
- 1/2 teaspoon cayenne pepper
- 1-2 tablespoons extra virgin olive oil
- 12 ounces chicken stock
- 1/2 cup orange juice
- Corn tortillas

- Avocado slices
- 2% plain Greek yogurt
- Fresh cilantro
- Hot sauce
- Lime wedges
- Salsa

Method

1. Preheat oven to 175 degrees C. Mix together all of the spices in a small bowl. Coat the pork pieces with the spice mixture.

2. Heat the oil in a big pot over medium-high heat. Add the pork; cook for 1 minute on each side. Remove the meat from the heat, and set it aside for later.

3. Pour in the chicken stock and orange juice, and bring everything to a boil. Add the pork back to the pot. Cover the pot, and place it in the oven for about 30 minutes to keep it warm.

4. Remove the pot form the oven to flip the pork pieces. Return it to the oven (without a lid) for about 1-½ hours, flipping the pork occasionally to make sure it cooks evenly.

5. When it's finished cooking, shred the pork in the pot, mix it with the sauce until everything is incorporated. Serve the pork with hot sauce, cilantro, lime, or salsa.

Dinner: Sealed Hake with Olive Salsa

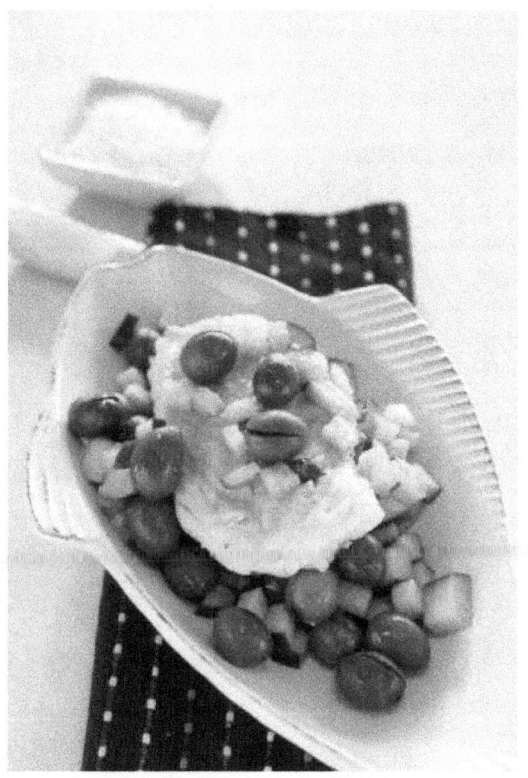

Ingredients

- 4 hake fillets
- 2 tablespoons melted margarine
- 1 cup black olives
- 1 cup thinly sliced cucumber
- ¼ cup oil
- 1½ tablespoon vinegar
- Salt and pepper to taste

Method

1. Heat the pan on medium-high heat.

2. Meanwhile, brush the fillets with the margarine and season them with salt and pepper to taste. Fry hake for 7 minutes on each side.

3. Mix olives and cucumber in a bowl, and sprinkle them with oil and vinegar. Season well and serve with salsa.

Snacks: Whole Wheat Toast with Peanut Butter & A Fruit Smoothie

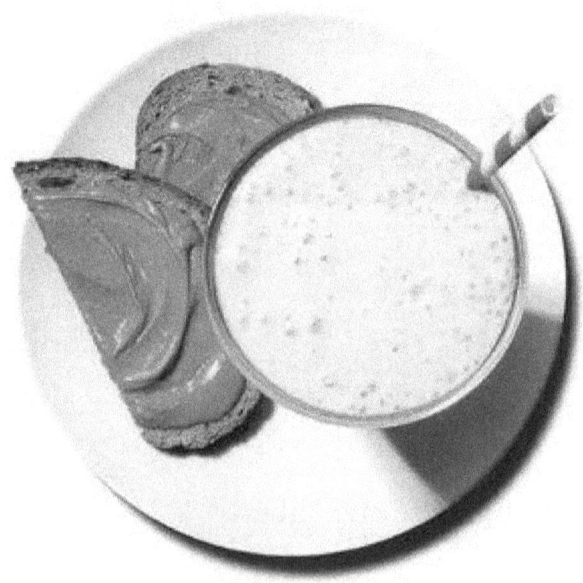

See Week 1 Day 1 For Smoothie Recipe

Others who are considering purchasing this book would love to know what you think. If you could spare a few seconds, they would greatly appreciate reading an honest review from you. Simply visit the page on Amazon.com.

Week 4

Day 5

Breakfast: Boiled Egg with Strawberries

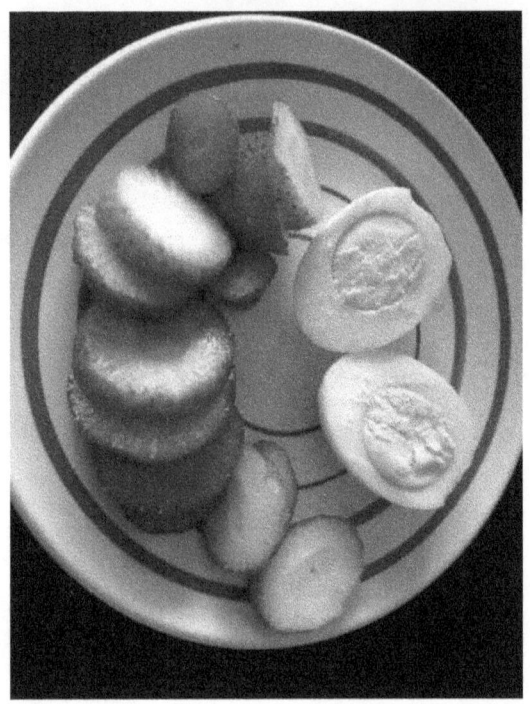

Ingredients

- 1 cup of skim milk
- 1 boiled egg
- A handful of fresh strawberries
- 1 piece of toast

Method

1. Bring a pot of water to a boil. Add 1 tablespoon of vinegar. Carefully crack the egg into the boiling water, pushing the whites toward the yolk with a metal spoon.

2. Allow the egg to cook for several minutes until it reaches desired firmness.

3. Remove the egg with a slotted spoon. Enjoy with strawberries and a piece of whole-wheat toast.

Lunch: Fresh Fruit Salad

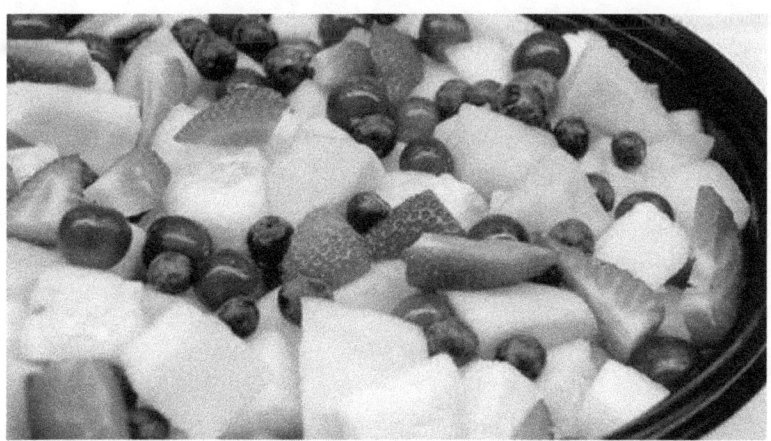

Ingredients

- 1 bowl of fruits of your choice (cubed)
- Pepper (a pinch)
- Juice of one lemon

Method

1. Add a pinch of pepper and lemon to the fruit. Enjoy!

Dinner: Slow Cooked Thai Curry Beef with Whole Wheat Pasta

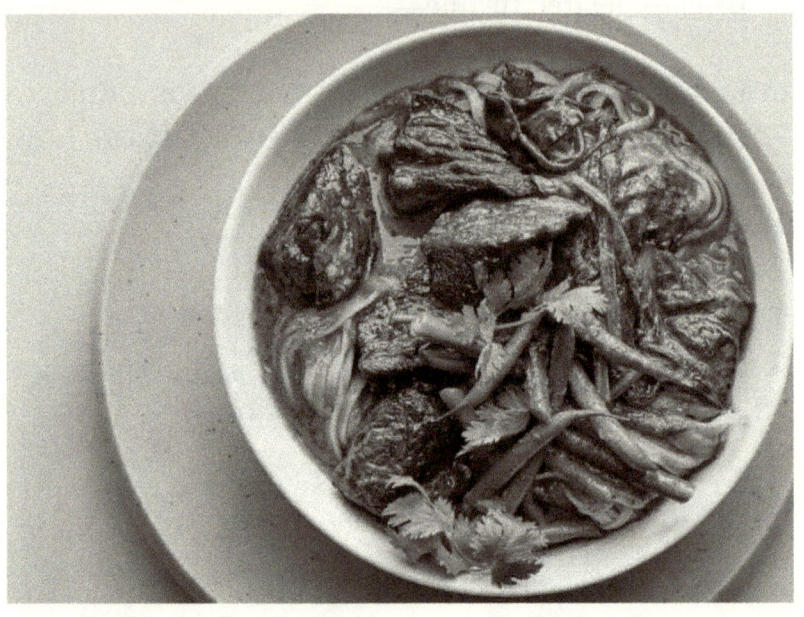

See Week 1 Day 5 For Recipe

Snacks: Apple, Roasted Peanuts, & Raisins

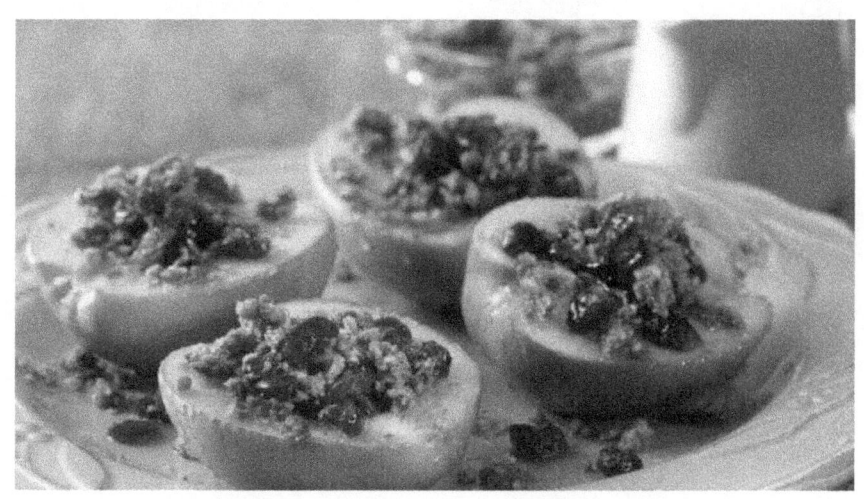

Week 4

Day 6

Breakfast: Boiled Oats

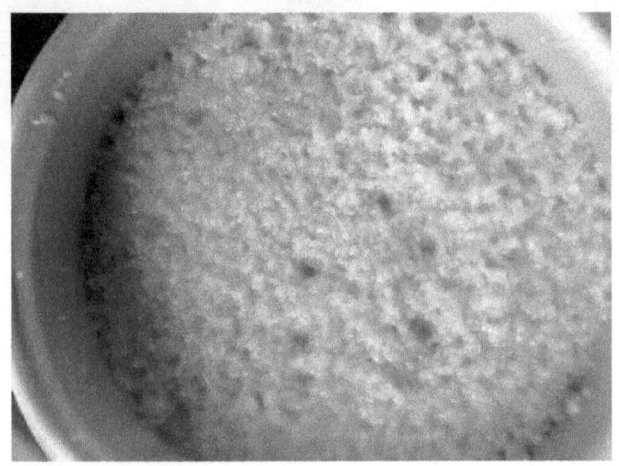

See Week 1 Day 4 For Recipe

Lunch: Lime Chicken, Black Beans, & Brown Rice

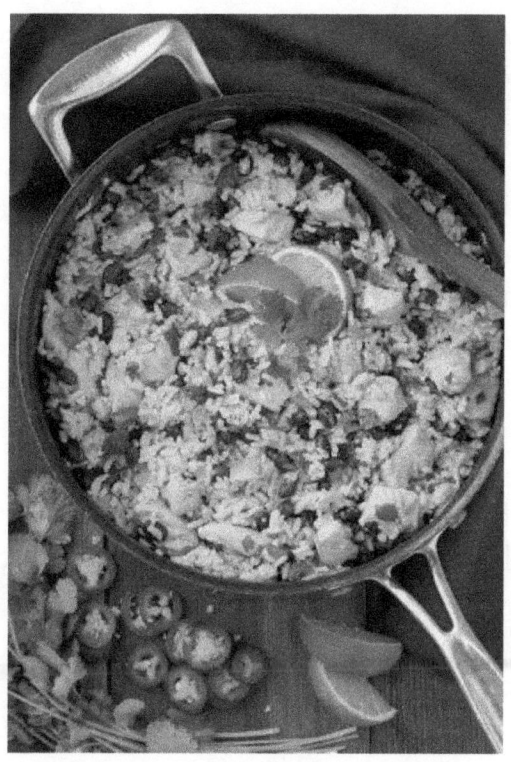

Ingredients

- 6 tablespoons honey
- 6 tablespoons soy sauce (low sodium if available)
- 2 teaspoons lime zest
- 6 tablespoons lime juice
- 1 teaspoon crushed red pepper
- 4 chicken thighs
- 2 chicken breasts

Method

1. Mix together all ingredients except the chicken.

2. Put the chicken in a deep bowl and coat it in the mixture. Place the bowl in the fridge for at least two hours (or overnight to marinate).

3. Preheat a grill to 200 degrees C. (You can also use a charcoal grill, but move all the charcoals to one side and cook the chicken on the other side.)

4. Remove the chicken from the marinade, and cook the marinade for 8-10 minutes until it starts to thicken.

5. Place the chicken on the grill and cook for 8-10 minutes on each side, and glaze periodically with the marinade. Serve with black beans and brown rice.

Dinner: Sweet & Sour Pork

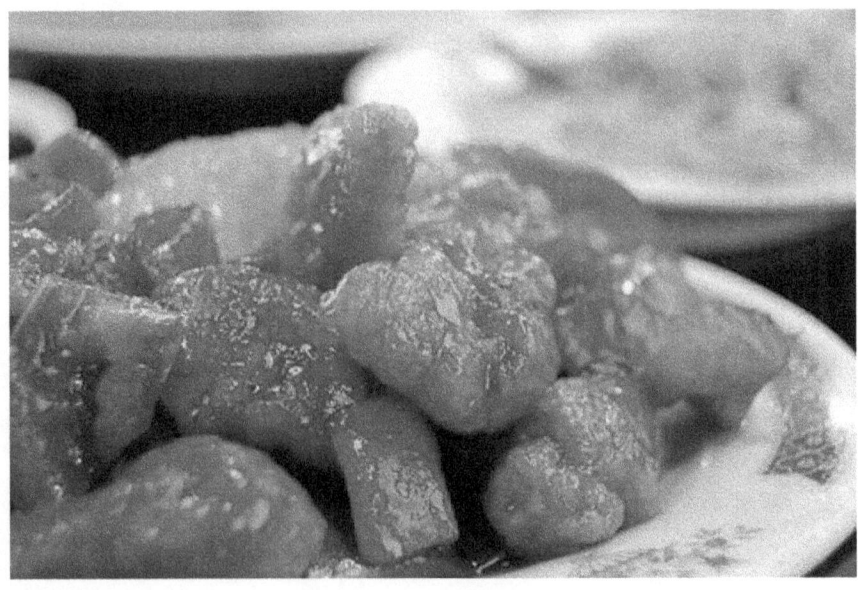

Ingredients

- ¼ cup olive oil
- 1 tablespoon minced fresh ginger
- 18 ounces cubed pork all fat trimmed
- 1 tablespoon soy sauce
- 2 tablespoons sweet chili sauce
- 1 cup canned pineapple (drained)
- 1 red pepper (cubed)
- 2 sliced spring onions
- Pepper to taste

Method

1. Heat the oil over medium heat until it is very hot. Add the ginger, and cook for 3 minutes until fragrant. Add the pork, and cook for 4 minutes.

2. Add the rest of the ingredients, and cook for another 3-4 minutes. Season well, and serve with boiled potatoes.

Snacks: Fresh Fruit, Peanuts, & Raisins

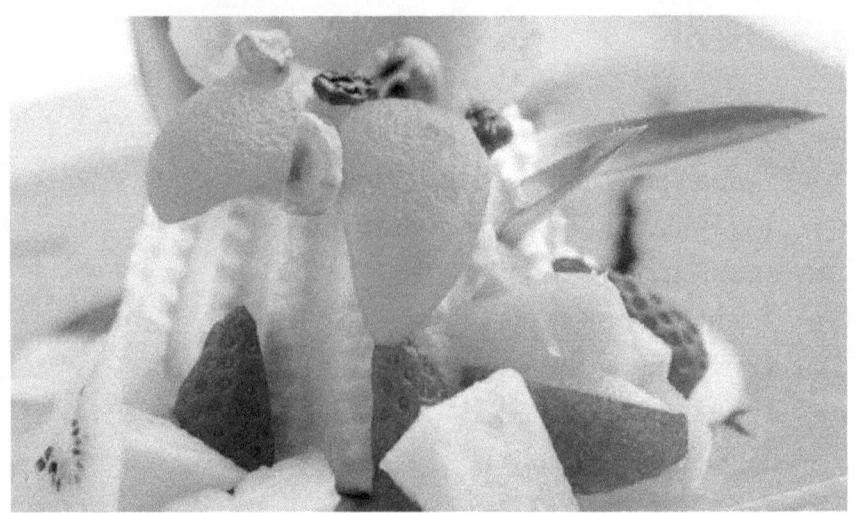

Week 4

Day 7

Breakfast: Homemade Yogurt

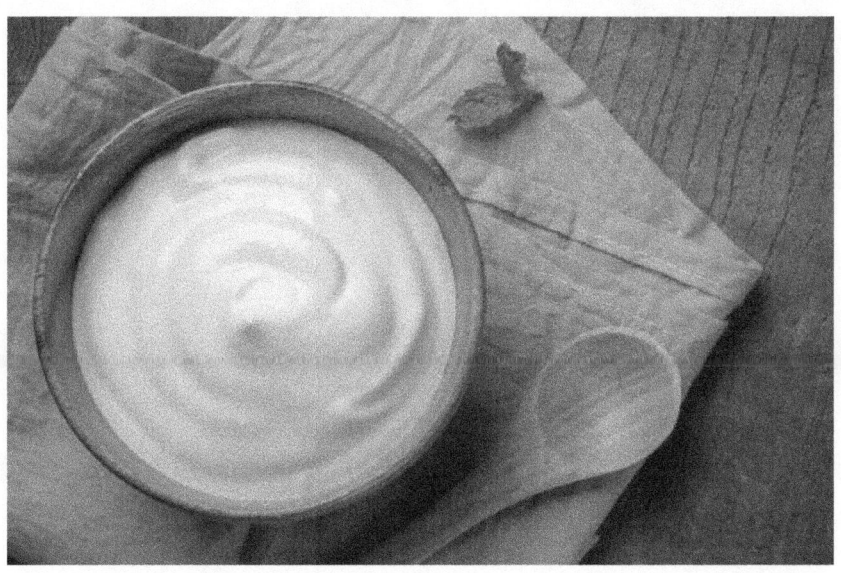

See Week 2 Day 1 For Recipe

Lunch: Avocado Chicken Salad

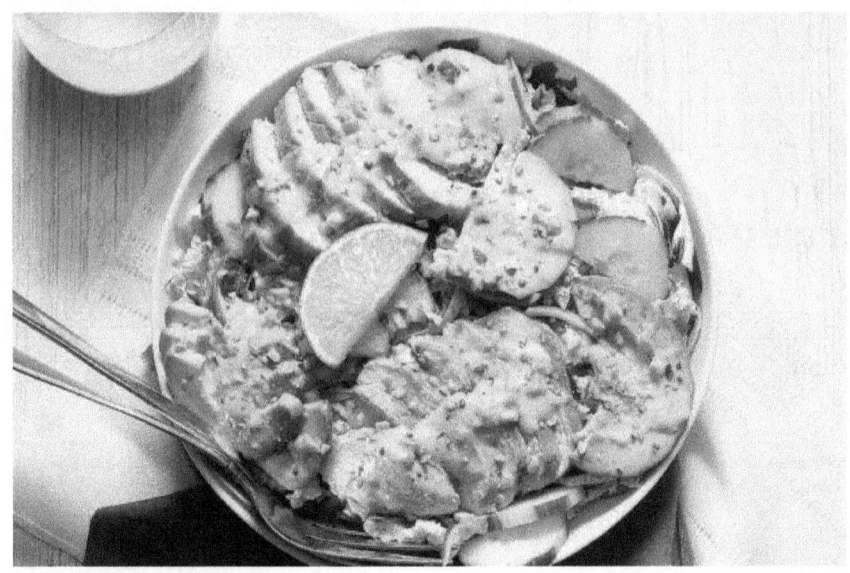

Ingredients

- ½ red onion, chopped
- 1 small lime
- 1 avocado
- ½ teaspoon onion powder
- ¼ teaspoon salt
- ¼ ground pepper
- ½ cup plain Greek yogurt
- ½ teaspoon garlic
- 2 cups cooked chicken (either chopped or shredded)

Method

1. Mash together the avocado and Greek yogurt until they are smooth.

2. Stir in all of the spices. Add the chicken and onion to the bowl, and coat in the mixture.

3. Squeeze in the lime juice to taste. Eat the chicken salad in a wrap or on its own.

Dinner: Rosemary Lamb Chops

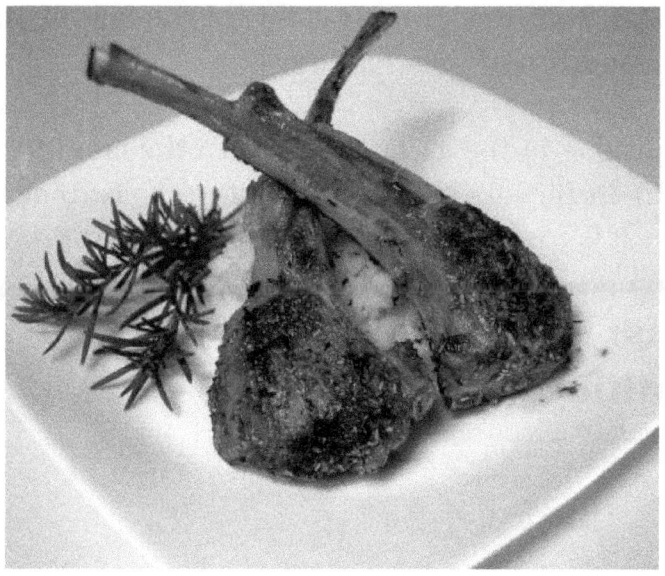

Ingredients

- 18 ounces pork chops
- 1 tablespoon flour
- 2 teaspoon dried rosemary
- 3 tablespoon olive oil
- 9 ounces sliced mushrooms
- Finely chopped garlic clove
- 1 ½ cups of vegetable stock

Method

1. Cut the lamb into thin strips. Mix the rosemary, flour, salt, and pepper in a bowl. Coat the lamb strips in this mixture.

2. Heat 2 tablespoons of oil in a wide frying pan, and fry the lamb until it is browned on both sides. Remove the meat from the pan. Heat the remaining oil, and cook the mushrooms for 2 minutes.

3. Sprinkle in the garlic, and return the lamb to the pan. Stir in the stock until the mixture boils. Simmer until meat is cooked. Serve with couscous or brown rice.

Snacks: Any Citrus Fruit & A Kale Apple Smoothie

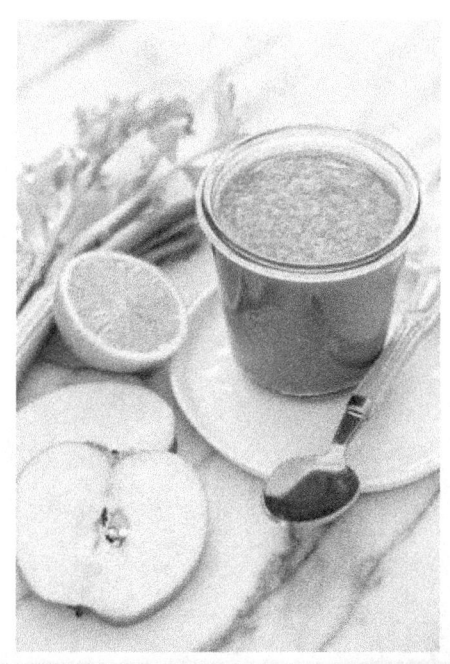

See Week 2 Day 2 For Recipe

Week 5

Day 1

Breakfast: Chicken Sausage & Egg Slow Cooker Casserole

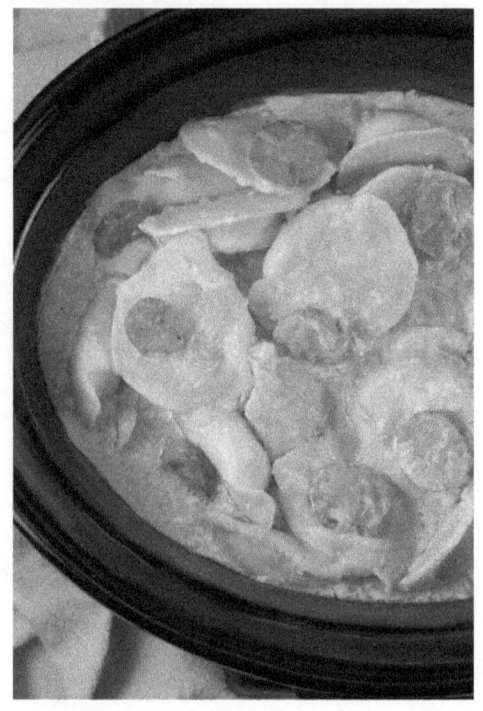

See Week 1 Day 3 For Recipe

Lunch: Overstuffed Vegetable Sandwich

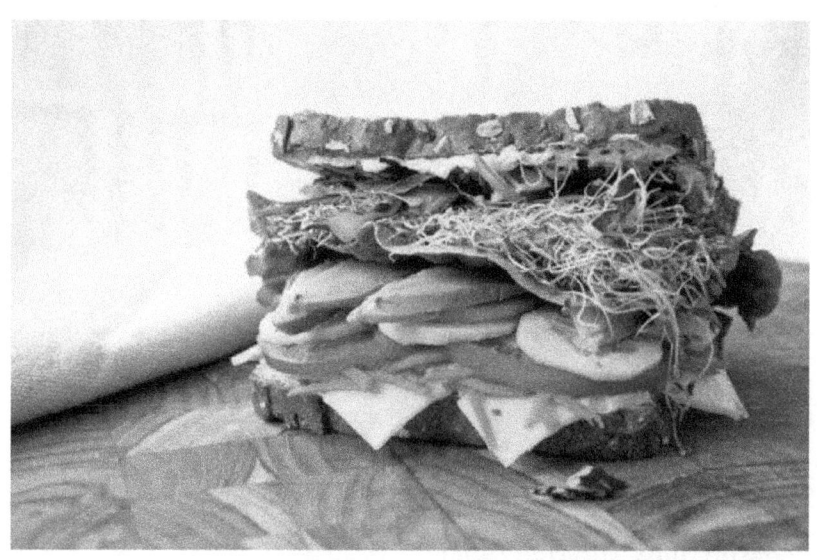

See Week 3 Day 1 For Recipe

Dinner: Sautéed Asparagus with Grilled Fish

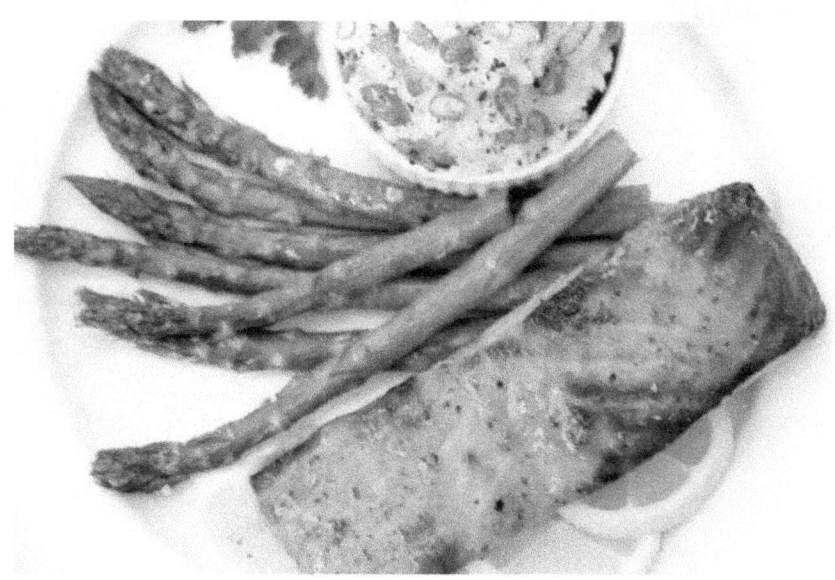

Ingredients

- ½ Pound fish fillets
- 1 teaspoon lemon juice
- ½ teaspoon garlic powder
- Salt and pepper to taste
- Sautéed Asparagus (for the side)

Method

1. Combine the lemon, garlic powder, salt, and pepper. Marinate the fish in the mixture.

2. Grill for 2-3 minutes on each side. Serve with sautéed asparagus.

Snacks: Any Citrus Fruit & A Kale Apple Smoothie

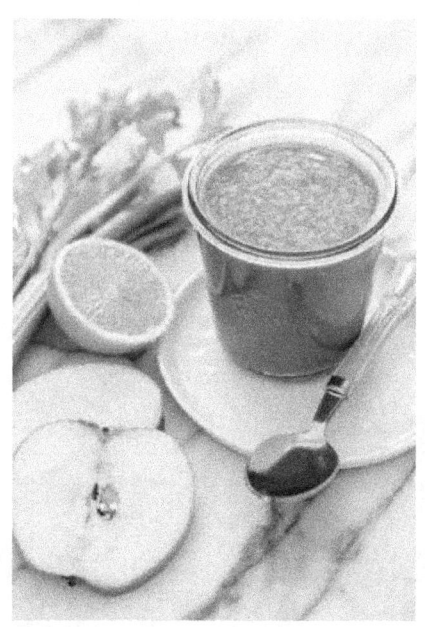

See Week 2 Day 2 For Recipe

Week 5

Day 2

Breakfast: Tofu Scramble

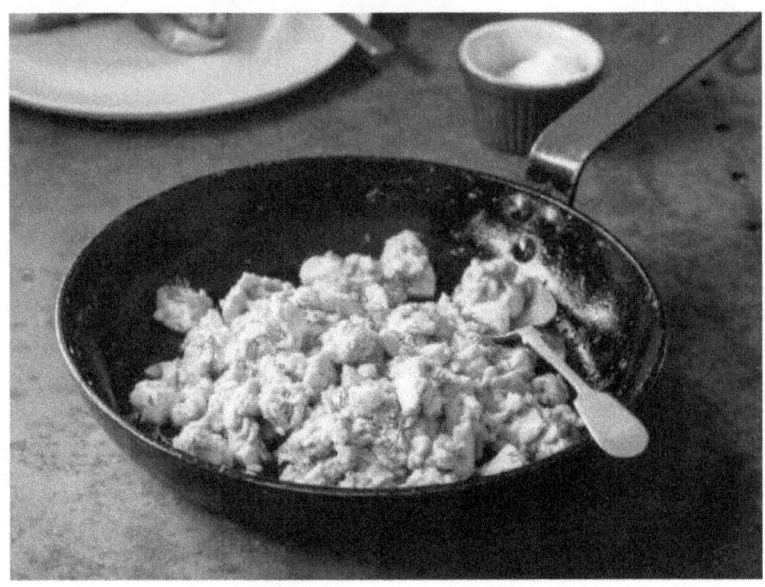

See Week 1 Day 5 For Recipe

Lunch: Tomato Risotto with Rosemary & Basil

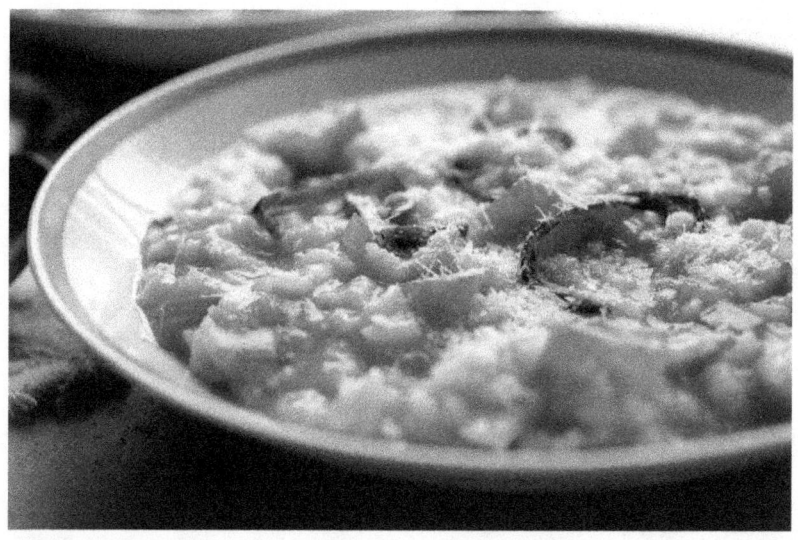

Ingredients

- 1 cup risotto rice
- 1 1/3 cups cherry tomatoes (halved)
- Small pack basil (roughly torn)
- 4 tablespoons grated parmesan
- 1 ½ cups chopped tomatoes
- 1 ½ cups vegetable stock
- 1 tablespoon of butter
- 1 tablespoon olive oil
- 1 onion (finely chopped)
- 2 garlic cloves (finely chopped)
- 1 rosemary sprig (finely chopped)

Method

1. Make a mixture of vegetable stock, tomatoes, rosemary, and basil in a processor.

2. Soften onions in butter, and then add garlic and the above mixture slowly.

3. Let the risotto cook until it's creamy. Serve with the parmesan on top.

Dinner: Traditional Asian Chickpea Salad

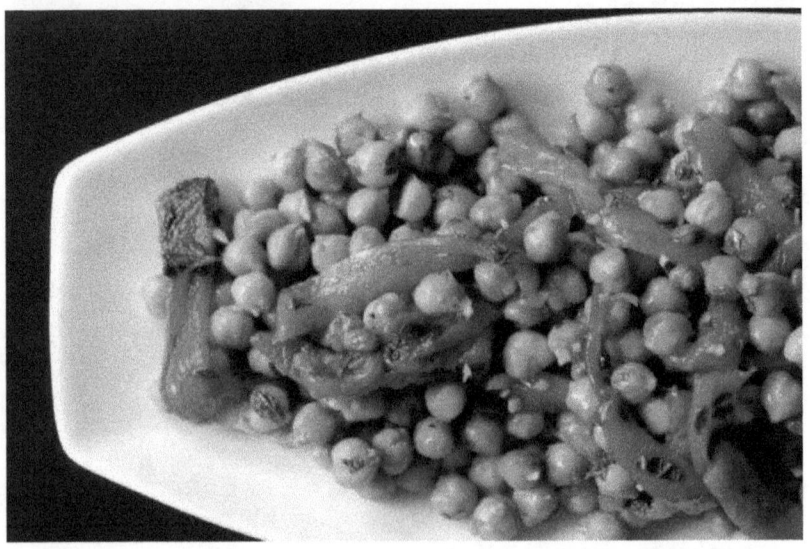

Ingredients

- 1 can chickpeas (drained and rinsed)
- Red chili flakes to your taste
- Salt to taste
- Juice of 1 lemon

Method

1. Mix all the ingredients in a bowl. Serve with chopped tomatoes and onions.

Snacks: Whole Wheat Toast with Peanut Butter & A Fruit Smoothie

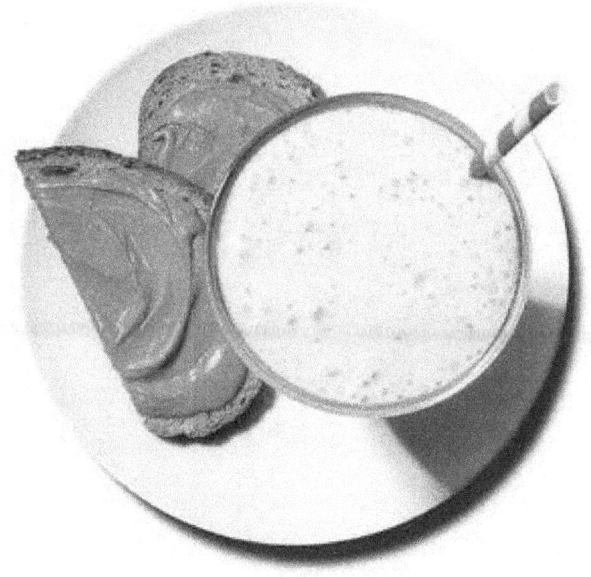

See Week 1 Day 1 For Smoothie Recipe

Don't forget to share your thoughts on this book by leaving a review on Amazon.com. It takes just a few seconds.

Week 5

Day 3

Breakfast: Low Fat Mango Yogurt

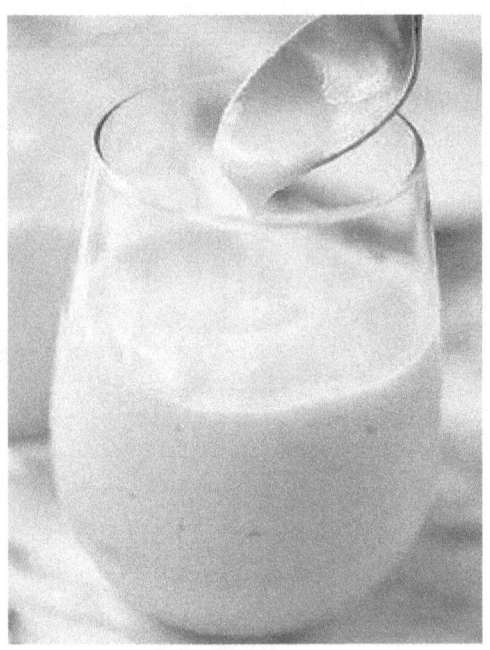

Ingredients

- 1 package low-fat yogurt
- 1 mango (cubed)
- 1 teaspoon low-fat cream

Method

1. Mix all the ingredients together until they form a consistent mixture. Let it set in the fridge for several hours (until firm).

Lunch: Grilled Prawns & Brown Rice

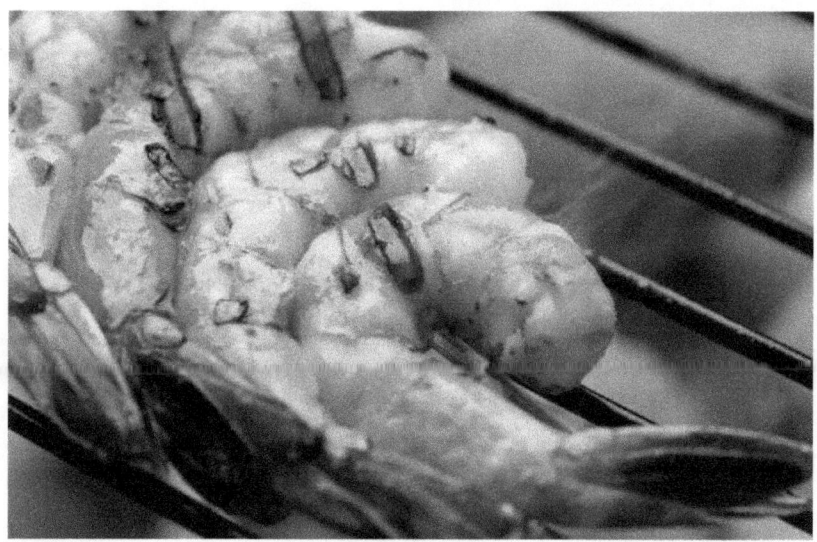

Ingredients

- 6 prawns
- Brown rice (cooked)
- Salt and pepper to taste
- Oregano
- Olive oil for grilling

Method

1. Heat oil in a skillet until it is very hot. Add in the prawns, and grill several minutes on each side. Season with salt and pepper to taste.

2. Toss brown rice with a dash of olive oil, salt, and oregano. Serve with green chutney!

Dinner: Roasted Tomatoes with Chickpeas

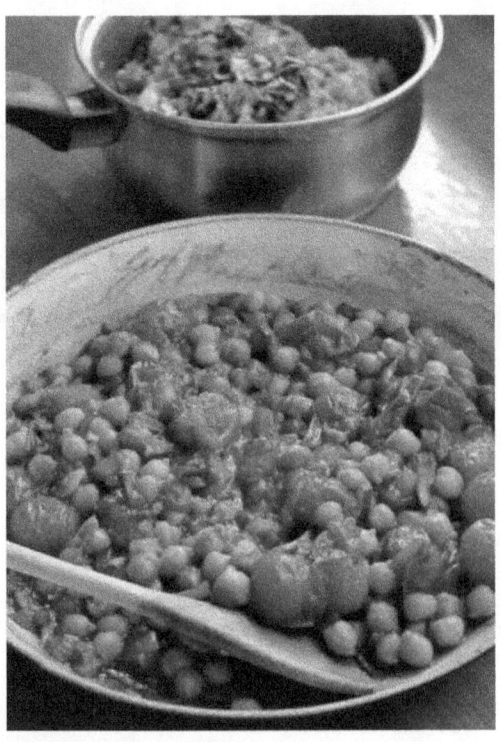

Ingredients

- 3-4 small red tomatoes (cut in half)
- 2 cloves grated garlic

- Salt and pepper to taste
- 1 can of chickpeas (strained and rinsed)
- 1/2 tablespoon lime juice
- Olive oil as required

Method

1. Heat the olive oil and grated garlic on medium heat until fragrant. Add in the tomatoes, and cook for 1 minute on both sides. Then plate the tomatoes.

2. Toss the chickpeas with lemon juice and a pinch of salt. Serve tomatoes on a bed of chickpeas. Garnish with oregano, if needed.

Snacks: Fruit Smoothie and a Fresh Vegetable

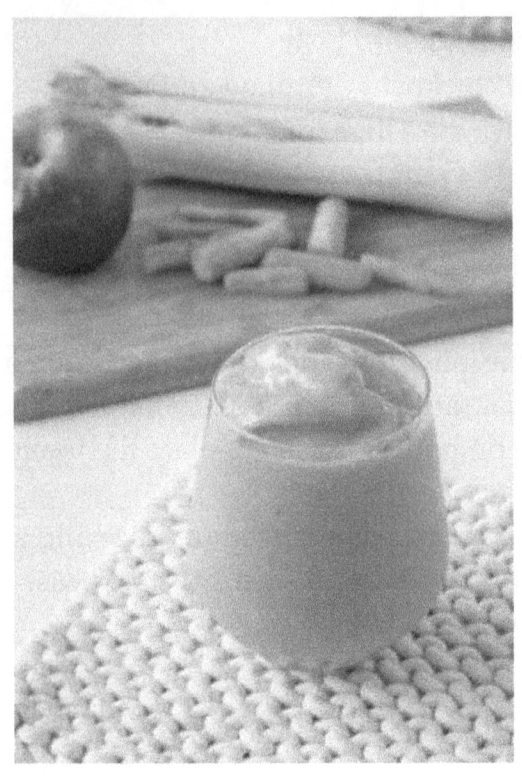

See Week 1 Day 1 For Recipe

Discover Scientifically-Proven "Shortcuts" & "Hacks" to Lose Weight FASTER (With Very Little Effort)

For this month only, you can get Linda's best-selling & most popular book absolutely free – *Weight Loss Secrets You NEED to Know*.

Get Your FREE Copy Here:
TopFitnessAdvice.com/Bonus

Discover scientifically-proven tips to help you lose weight faster and easier than ever before. With this book, readers were able to improve their weight loss results and fitness levels. So, it's highly recommended that you get this book, especially while it's free!

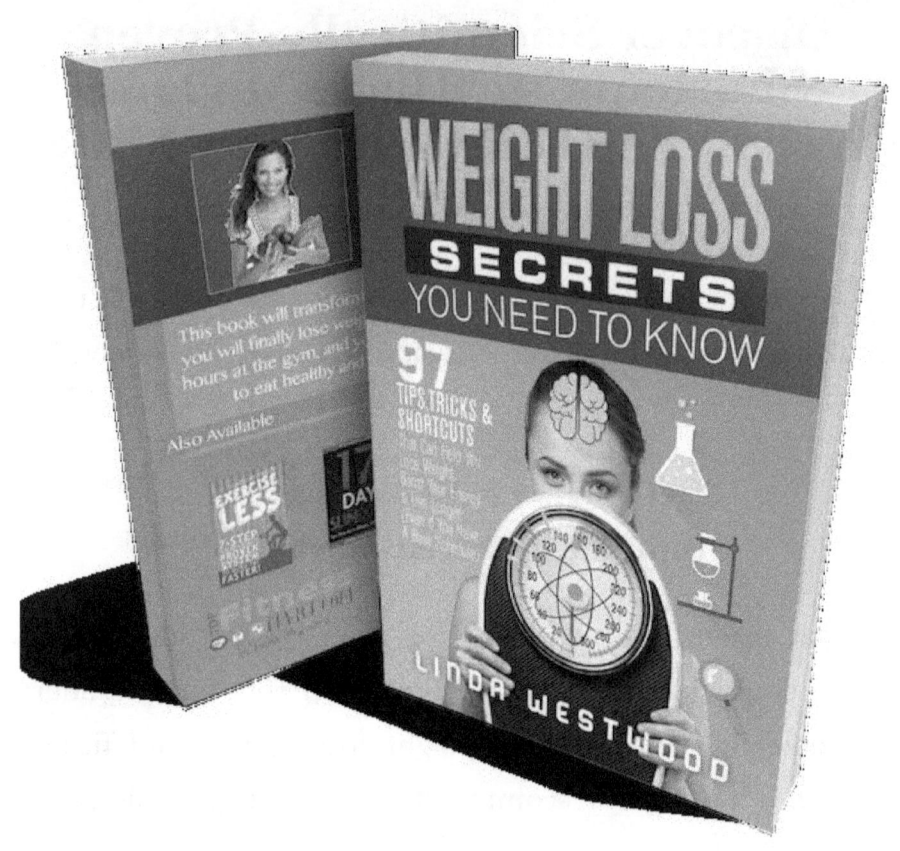

Get Your FREE Copy Here:
TopFitnessAdvice.com/Bonus

Final Words

I would like to thank you for purchasing my book and I hope I have been able to help you and educate you on something new.

If you have enjoyed this book and would like to share your positive thoughts, could you please take 30 seconds of your time to go back and give me a review on my Amazon book page.

I greatly appreciate seeing these reviews because it helps me share my hard work.

You can leave me a review on Amazon.com.

Again, thank you and I wish you all the best!

Enjoying this book?

Check out my other best sellers!

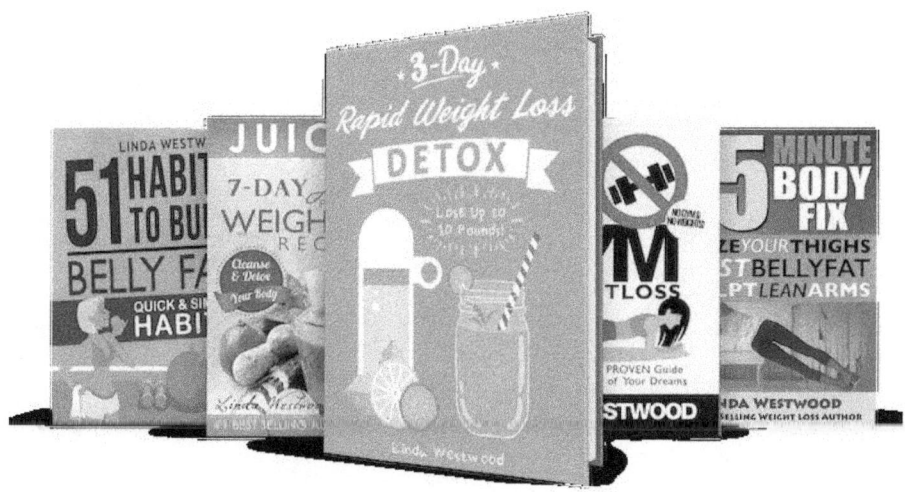

Get your next book on sale here:

TopFitnessAdvice.com/go/books

www.ingramcontent.com/pod-product-compliance
Lightning Source LLC
Chambersburg PA
CBHW031152020426
42333CB00013B/634